ACID-RELATED DISORDERS

George Sachs, MB., ChB., DSc.
UCLA
Los Angeles, California

Christian K. Prinz, M.D.
Second Department of Medicine
Universität München

Stephen J. Hersey, Ph.D.
Emory University
Atlanta, Ga.

Computer Illustrations
Steven M. Lustig, BioDesign

ACID-RELATED DISORDERS

Mystery to Mechanism:
Mechanism to Management

◁Sushu Publishing, Inc.

Design and Production
Maria S. Karkucinski
   Book Design Studio

Manuscript Editor
Andrew Kiburis

Indexer
Ed Yaeger

Library of Congress Cataloging-in-Publication Data

Acid related disorders: Mystery to mechanism: Mechanism to management / George Sachs,
   Christian K. Prinz, Stephen J. Hersey.
Includes bibliographical references and index.

ISBN 0-9639943-0-1

Library of Congress Catalog Number 95-67941 CIP

© SUSHU Communications, Inc. 1995

Distributed by SUSHU Communications Inc.

Sponsored by an unrestricted grant from Astra Merck. Astra Merck did not influence the content or distribution of this text book and will not profit from its distribution.

Printed in the United States.

First published in 1995.

Contents

Preface

The secretion of hydrochloric acid by the stomach has been the subject of biological and clinical investigation for over a century. Gastric acid secretion presents a twofold challenge for medical science. From a biological perspective there is a desire to understand how the stomach can secrete a concentrated acid solution, namely the mechanism of acid secretion, while from a clinical perspective there is a need to treat disorders which are associated with this acid solution, namely the management of acid secretion. Given this dual challenge, it is not surprising that improvements in the management of acid-related disorders have evolved together with an improved understanding of the mechanism of acid secretion.

While there is much yet to be learned, our understanding of the mechanism of gastric acid secretion has progressed rapidly and at an accelerated pace over the last decade. This knowledge allows for a more precise appreciation of the mechanisms of action and limitations of current therapeutic anti-secretory agents as well as providing the prospect of rational design of future therapeutic approaches to acid-related disorders.

This publication is organized in keeping with the mechanisms and management of gastric acid secretion. Following a brief historical perspective, we present a current view of the mechanism of acid secretion (Section I) and the factors which regulate this process (Section II). Emphasis here is on the most recent developments and those aspects which relate directly to therapeutic control of acid secretion. The mechanism of action of anti-secretory agents is presented in light of our current concepts of acid secretion (Section III). Subsequently, the clinical use of these agents for symptom relief and management of acid-related disorders is described (Section IV). Finally, Section V deals with possible future trends in therapy of acid-related diseases, emphasizing the emerging role of *Helicobacter pylori*. We have not attempted to provide complete and detailed coverage of these subjects but have concentrated on the most recent developments and cited only selected references due to space limitations.

We hope that this publication will provide a rapid update for those already familiar with the area as well as an initial reference source for those wishing to obtain more detailed information on gastric acid secretion and its clinical management. To accomplish these goals each section of the book has an overview summarizing the section, and is immediately followed by figures with explanatory legends. These are followed by a more detailed text explaining the concepts involved in the fascinating physiological and biochemical process of acid secretion and its pharmacological control.

GEORGE SACHS, MB. ,ChB., DSc.
UCLA, Los Angeles, Ca.

CHRISTIAN K. PRINZ, M.D.
Second Department of Medicine, Universität München.

STEPHEN J. HERSEY, Ph.D.
Emory University, Atlanta, Ga.

Introduction

Advances over the past two decades have revolutionized our concepts of acid secretion and its management in acid-related disorders. Most of this publication is directed at those recent developments. These advances have evolved from a substantial base of scientific and clinical investigation extending over the last 200 years or more and may best be appreciated within the context of a historical perspective. As an introduction to the following sections we present here a brief history of gastric acid secretion and its clinical management.

Gastric Acid Secretion

Acid secretion by the stomach is a universal attribute of all vertebrates. This physiological process represents one element in a complex system which allows higher organisms to regulate their nutritional intake. Gastric acid aids digestion of food by allowing activity of the acid proteinase pepsin, helps to kill prey that is ingested live, and helps to sterilize the gastric contents. Hippocrates is credited with the first recorded speculation on the function of the stomach, suggesting that it 'cooked' the food. The modern concept that the stomach digests, rather than cooks, food was demonstrated by de Réaumur in 1752 (1) when he placed containers of meat in the stomachs of birds and found that the meat was digested. Some thirty years later Spallanzani (2) showed that digestion was accomplished by the gastric juice and did not require a 'vital force'. The digestive function of the gastric juice was firmly established in the nineteenth century following the demonstration by Prout (3) that the gastric juice contained muriatic acid, i.e., HCl, and the discovery of a gastric 'ferment' by Schwann, who named this enzyme pepsin (4). Subsequently, Langley (5) showed that the acid environment of the stomach is essential for the proteolytic activity of pepsin, establishing the need for both acid and pepsin in the digestive process. Langley also is credited with identifying the gastric chief cell as being responsible for the synthesis and secretion of pepsin.

The cellular origin of gastric acid was initially suggested in 1833 by Beaumont (6), who observed 'bright dots' on the lining of the stomach in his patient, Alexis St. Martin, who had a gastric fistula resulting from an accidental gunshot. Beaumont surmised that the dots were openings of secretory glands. The specific cell responsible for acid secretion was identified in 1893 by Golgi (7), who described an expansion of the secretory canaliculus of stimulated parietal cells. Although Golgi was able to document the canalicular expansion with remarkable accuracy, the actual presence of acid within the canaliculus was not confirmed until almost a century later (figure 1).

During the first half of the twentieth century investigations of gastric acid production centered primarily on the mechanisms which control secretion. Pavlov (8) described in detail the 'cephalic phase' of secretory regulation in his classic studies in dogs and applied the principles of conditioning to show the presence of a 'psychic' or higher level of regulation. Central stimulation of acid secretion was shown to be mediated solely by the vagus nerve, an observation on which was based the widespread use of vagotomy as an anti-secretory therapy.

The existence of peripheral stimulatory mechanisms was proposed by Edkins in 1905 (9), when he demonstrated that an extract from the gastric antrum could stimulate acid secretion. Edkins termed the active principle in this extract 'gastrin'. However, the discovery of histamine in intestinal mucosa by Barger and Dale in 1911 (10), coupled to the demonstration by Popielski in 1920 (11) that histamine stimulates acid secretion, led to the erroneous conclusion that gastrin and histamine are the same. Some twenty years later, Komarov (12) demonstrated that gastrin is distinct from histamine, and in 1964 Gregory and Tracy isolated gastrin from the gastric antrum and characterized it as a peptide hormone (13). While these investigations firmly identified gastrin as a hormonal stimulant of acid secretion, they did not define its mechanism of action, a matter which remains controversial. Further, the stimulatory effect of histamine set the stage for one of the major historical controversies surrounding gastric function, namely, whether there is a final 'common' pathway of stimulation of acid secretion or whether gastrin, acetylcholine, and histamine are all direct stimulants of the parietal cell. A partial answer to this question became available in the 1970's when James Black and his co-workers developed anti-histamines selective for gastric acid secretion, the H_2 receptor antagonists (14). These antagonists were found to inhibit acid secretion stimulated, not only by histamine, but also by gastrin, acetylcholine, and ingestion of food. Thus histamine was shown to be a major endogenous stimulant. Moreover, the finding suggested that histamine acts as a common mediator for stimulation by gastrin and acetylcholine. Recent investigations of enterochromaffin-like cells, the histamine-releasing cells of the gastric mucosa, may provide a definitive answer in this controversy.

FIG. 1. A camera lucida drawing as published by Camillo Golgi, showing the canaliculus of the resting parietal cell on the left and the canaliculus of the stimulated parietal cell on the right. The expanded appearance, following stimulation, allowed him to conclude, 100 years ago, that the parietal cell's canaliculus was the source of acid in the stomach.

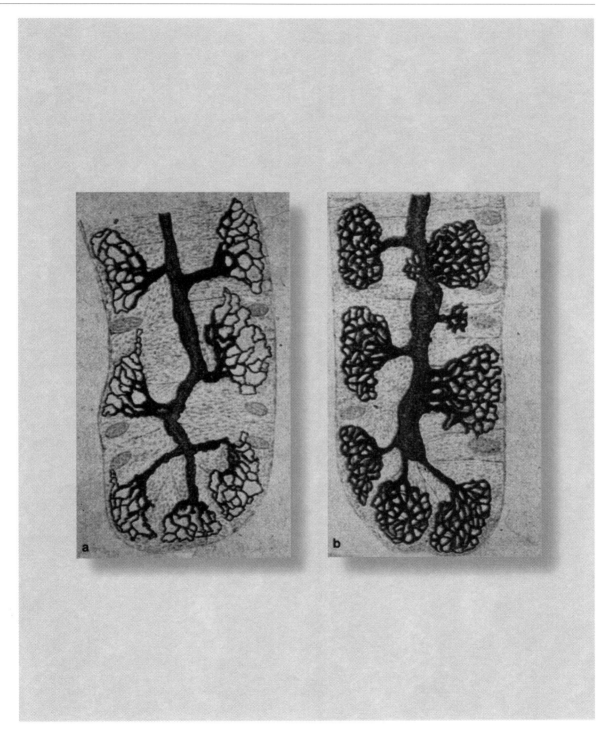

FIG. 1

Beginning in the 1960's the development of functional cellular and subcellular model systems permitted rapid progress in defining the cellular and molecular basis for acid secretion by the gastric parietal cell. Early hypotheses for the mechanism of acid secretion derived from the original suggestion by Claude Bernard (15) that the stomach secreted a precursor substance which was converted to acid in the stomach lumen. This erroneous suggestion resulted in a fruitless search for the precursor which lasted nearly eighty years. In the 1940's it was finally accepted that water is the only substance which could supply sufficient protons to account for the observed rate of gastric acid production (16). Investigations then centered on defining the energetic mechanism by which the parietal cell separated H^+ from OH^-. Two general mechanisms were in vogue in the 1950's, a redox mechanism and a high-energy organic phosphate mechanism. The redox mechanism was based on the known ability of redox enzymes in mitochondria to separate protons from electrons, and a similar mechanism had been proposed to account for anion accumulation by the roots of plants (17). Accordingly, this hypothesis suggested a separation of electrons and hydrogen ions across the secretory membrane, with the electrons being accepted by a cytoplasmic oxidant, the protons excreted as acid (16). Although such a mechanism was recognized correctly by Peter Mitchell as responsible for generating the proton gradient or proton motive force across the mitochondrial, chloroplast, and bacterial membrane necessary for the synthesis of ATP (18), it has proved incorrect for gastric acid formation. The alternative mechanism proposed that the chemical energy contained in the phosphate ester bonds of ATP could be used to transport hydrogen ions derived from water (16). The latter hypothesis was given significant support in 1957 when Jens Skou described an adenosine triphosphatase which he proposed to be the sodium pump (19). According to this proposal ATP, not redox reactions, provided the energy for sodium transport, and the sodium pump exchanged sodium for potassium. The demonstration of ATP-driven proton transport in gastric cell membranes (20) and the discovery and characterization of an enzyme, the H^+,K^+-ATPase, which utilizes the chemical energy of ATP to transport hydrogen ions out of the cell in exchange for potassium ions into the cell, illuminated the mechanism of gastric acid secretion (21,22). Over the past decade, substantial evidence has accumulated to identify the H^+,K^+-ATPase as the gastric acid pump. Molecular analysis of the H^+,K^+-ATPase has confirmed that this enzyme is similar to the sodium pump and quite distinct from the proton pump of mitochondria, thus settling the controversy over the molecular basis of gastric acid secretion. Moreover, the unique distribution and properties of the H^+,K^+-ATPase suggest that this enzyme could serve as a primary therapeutic target in acid-related disease.

■ Clinical Management

Dyspepsia has been recognized as a clinical entity since the dawn of medicine. The more severe forms of this disorder, including reflux esophagitis, gastric ulcer, and duodenal ulcer, have come to be universally associated with the presence of gastric acid secretion. Hence Schwartz's therapeutic dictum 'no acid no ulcer' (23) remains the basis of managing these disorders. While the incidence of acid-related disorders, at one time or another in life, is about 20% of the population (male or female), everyone secretes acid throughout life. It remains a mystery which additional factors, in addition to acid, contribute to the development of disorders in a given individual. Recent epidemiological data have shown that infection with a bacterium, *Helicobacter pylori*, is also a requirement for the occurrence of duodenal ulcer and non-NSAID-induced gastric ulcer. The bacterium appears to play no role in esophagitis. Although a majority of the elderly are infected with *H. pylori* and secrete acid, only a minority develop peptic ulcer disease. However, in spite of our relative ignorance of the precise etiology of acid-related disorders, control of acid secretion alone is able to relieve the symptoms and promote healing of peptic ulcers, and eradication of *H. pylori* can apparently cure peptic ulcer disease.

A variety of therapies, both surgical and medical, designed to reduce acid secretion have evolved over the past century, ablating either stimulation or production of acid. In the late nineteenth century, the Viennese surgeon Christian Billroth introduced total or partial gastric resection to remove the acid-secreting portion of the stomach. Variations of this surgical procedure persisted as a primary treatment for ulcer disease well into this century. Vagotomy, introduced by Latarjet in 1922 (24) and reintroduced by Dragstedt in 1943 (25), became one of the most frequent operations for peptic ulcer following its combination with antrectomy by Smithwick (26). Selective vagotomy, denervating only the stomach, was developed in 1948, and some 20 years later highly selective vagotomy, namely denervation of only the proximal fundic gland area of the stomach, was introduced into surgical practice. The major pharmacological approach to ulcer disease prior to the 1970's was the use of atropine, extracted from berries of a plant, deadly nightshade. The vagal pathway of acid secretory stimulation is the site of action of this drug. Thus the first three quarters of the twentieth century was the era of the vagus in terms of clinical management of acid-related disorders.

The synthesis and description of the actions of the H_2 histamine receptor antagonists by James Black in 1971 (14) heralded a new era in the medical treatment of acid-related disorders, the era of the parietal cell. The H_2 receptor antagonists acting on the basal surface of the parietal cell proved to be effective and well tolerated inhibitors of acid secretion, and their use has substantially reduced the need for surgical intervention. The individual variability of response to H_2 receptor antagonists, due to a variety of factors such as tolerance, acid rebound, and variation of stimulus pathways, has resulted in sub-optimal healing at standard doses for peptic ulcer and reflux esophagitis.

Thus a need for more effective acid inhibition for optimal healing prompted a continuing search for other pharmacological agents. This search resulted in the development of another class of anti-secretory agents, the acid pump inhibitors (27). These agents selectively target the parietal cell, are well tolerated by the majority of patients, and have few side effects. Unlike the H_2 receptor antagonists, however, acid pump inhibitors target the final step in acid secretion, the H^+,K^+-ATPase of the parietal cell, and therefore their action is selective and is independent of the intensity or nature of parietal cell stimulation. Phenomena such as tolerance and acid rebound are also not found with the pump inhibitors. This class of drug has been designed in order to replace the H_2 receptor antagonists as the mainstay of therapy of peptic ulcers and reflux disease.

REFERENCES

1. Réaumur, René, A. F. de: Sur la digestion des oiseaux. Mem. Acad. Roy. d. Sc. Paris, 1752, pp. 266.

2. Spallanzani, A. L.: Delle digestione degli animale. In Fisica animale, Venice, 1782.

3. Prout, W.: On the nature of the acid and saline matters usually existing in the stomach of animals. Philos. Trans. 114, 45, 1824.

4. Schwann, T.: Über das Wesen des Verdauungsprozessus. Mueller's Arch. Berlin, pp. 90, 1836.

5. Langley, J. N.: On the histology and physiology of pepsin-forming glands. Phil. Trans. Roy. Soc. Lond. Ser. B 172, 664, 1881.

6. Beaumont, W.: Experiments and Observations on the Gastric Juice and the Physiology of Digestion. Plattsburg, F. P. Allen, 1833.

7. Golgi, C.: Sur la fine organisation des glandes peptiques des mammifères. Arch. Ital. Biol. 19, 448, 1893.

8. Pavlov, I.: The Work of the Digestive Glands. English translation from the Russian by W. H. Thompson, London, C. Griffin and Co., 1910.

9. Edkins, J. S.: On the chemical mechanism of gastric secretion. Proc. Roy. Soc. London. Ser. B 76, 376, 1905.

10. Barger, G. and Dale, H. H.: β-Imidazolyethylamine a depressor constituent of intestinal mucosa. J. Physiol. (London) 41, 499, 1911.

11. Popielski, L.: β-imidazolyaethylamin und die Orgunextrakte; β-imidazolyaethylamin als maechtiger Erreger der Magendruesen. Pflueger Arch. Ges. Physiol. 178, 214, 1920.

12. Komarov, S. A.: Gastrin. Proc. Soc. Exp. Biol. Med. 38, 514, 1938.

13. Gregory, R. A. and Tracy, H. J.: The constitution and properties of two gastrins extracted from hog antral mucosa. Gut 5, 103, 1964.

14. Black, J. W., Duncan, W. A. M., Durant, C. J., Ganellin, C. R., and Parsons, E. M.: Definition and antagonism of histamine H_2-receptors. Nature 236, 385, 1972.

15. Bernard, C.: Propriétés physiologiques des liquides de l'organisme. Paris, 1858.

16. Davies, R. E.: The mechanism of hydrochloric acid production by the stomach. Biol. Revs. 26, 87, 1951.

17. Lundegårdh, H.: Investigations as to the absorption and accumulation of inorganic ions. Ann. Agric. Coll. Sweden 8, 233, 1940.

18. Mitchell, P.: Chemiosmotic coupling in oxidative and photosynthetic phosphorylation. Biol. Rev. 41, 445, 1966.

19. Skou, J. C.: The influence of some cations on an adenosine triphosphatase from peripheral nerves. Biochim. Biophys. Acta 23, 394, 1957.

20. Lee, J., Simpson, G., and Scholes, P.: An ATPase from dog gastric mucosa, changes of outer pH in suspensions of dog membrane vesicles accompanying ATP hydrolysis. Biochem. Biophys. Res. Commun. 60, 825, 1974.

21. Ganser, A. L. and Forte, J.G.: K^+-stimulated ATPase in purified microsomes of bullfrog oxyntic cells. Biochim. Biophys. Acta 307, 169, 1973.

22. Sachs, G., Chang, H. H., Rabon E., Schackman, R., Lewin, M., and Saccomani, G.: A non-electrogenic H^+ pump in plasma membranes of hog stomach. J. Biol. Chem. 251, 7690, 1976.

23. Schwartz, K.: Ueber penetrierende Magen- und Jejunal Geschuere. Beitr. Klin. Chirurgie 5, 98, 1910.

24. Cade, A., and Latarjet, A.: Réalisation pathologique du petit estomac de Pavlov; Etude physiologique et histologique. J. Physiol. Path. Gén. 7, 221, 1905.

25. Dragstedt, L. R., and Owens, F. M., Jr.: Supradiaphragmatic section of the vagus nerves in treatment of duodenal ulcer. Proc. Soc. Exp. Biol. Med. 53, 125, 1943.

26. Smithwick, R. H., Harrower, H. W., and Farmer, D. A.: Hemigastrectomy and vagotomy in the treatment of duodenal ulcer. Am. J. Surg. 101, 325, 19.

27. Fellenius, E., Berglindh, T., Sachs, G., Olbe, L., Elander, B., Sjostrand, S. E., and Wallmark, B.: Substituted benzimidazoles inhibit gastric acid secretion by blocking H/K-ATPase. Nature 290, 159, 1981.

Mechanism of Acid Secretion

OVERVIEW

The gastric fundic epithelium is a monolayer, consisting of superficial surface mucus-secreting cells, and infoldings called gastric glands. These glands contain the neck or progenitor cells, and peptic (chief) and parietal cells. The parietal cell of the stomach has been identified as the cell responsible for secretion of gastric acid. Parietal cells are located in the oxyntic glands of the fundus and corpus of the stomach. A characteristic feature of the parietal cell is the presence of an invagination of the apical surface membrane known as the secretory canaliculus. Acid is secreted into the canaliculus and flows through this structure to the apical opening in the parietal cell surface and thence to the lumen of the oxyntic glands and to the lumen of the stomach.

The molecule responsible for secretion of gastric acid is an ATP-hydrolyzing enzyme, the gastric H^+,K^+-ATPase. This enzyme uses the chemical energy of ATP to transport protons from the cytoplasm of the parietal cell into the secretory canaliculi. The outward proton transport is accompanied by an inward transport of potassium so that one proton is exchanged for one potassium. The K^+ which is exchanged for H^+ enters the secretory canaliculi together with Cl^- by a passive transport mechanism from the cytoplasm of the parietal cell. The pump reabsorbs the K^+ in exchange for H^+ extrusion. The Cl^- remains with the H^+, resulting in the overall secretion of HCl.

The H^+,K^+- ATPase, the gastric acid pump, is found in large quantity only in the parietal cells of the stomach. It is only in this location that pH levels of about 1 are reached. The enzyme consists of two subunits. The larger, catalytic or α subunit, contains the ion binding sites and the catalytic activity of the enzyme. The smaller β subunit has no known direct enzymatic function but is necessary for stabilization of the conformation of the α subunit and, following biosynthesis, for targeting to the tubule membrane in the parietal cell. Both subunits are integral membrane proteins consisting of single chains of amino acids. The α subunit contains eight or ten regions or segments which span the membrane of the canaliculus, resulting in loops which project into the cytosol and extracellular space. It is therefore a polytopic integral membrane protein. The β subunit contains only one membrane-spanning region, and most of this protein projects into the secretory canaliculus. The extracellular surface of the β subunit is glycosylated. Together, these subunits form a functional transport unit capable of acid pumping.

2

When the parietal cell is not actively secreting acid, most of the H^+,K^+-ATPase is located in intracellular membrane organelles known as cytoplasmic tubules, and little is found in the secretory canaliculi. The acid pumps located in the tubules are inactive because the tubules are impermeable to K^+ and the H^+,K^+-ATPase cannot pump H^+ without K^+ at its outside surface. Stimulation of the parietal cell leads to conversion of the cytoplasmic tubules into the microvilli of the secretory canaliculi. This results in an expansion of the secretory canaliculi and allows most of the acid pumps to be present at the secretory surface. At the same time, the secretory surface becomes more permeable to K^+ and Cl^-, allowing the pumps present in the microvilli to become fully active, since K^+ is presented to the outside surface of the pump. When the stimulus is removed, the acid pump in the microvilli goes back to the tubules and the pumps become inactive. Even during maximal stimulation of the parietal cell, not all of the pumps are active, since there is a continual cycling of pumps into and out of the canaliculi. The intensity, nature and duration of stimulation determines the fraction of the acid pumps present in the secretory surface, and this factor together with the parietal cell mass determines the rate of gastric acid secretion.

The figures illustrating the mechanism of acid secretion are figures 2 through 17.

SITE OF ACID SECRETION
The Gastric Parietal Cell

Based on his observation that the surface invaginations of the parietal cell became enlarged during active secretion of acid, Golgi postulated in 1893 that this cell was the source of gastric acid (1). Further, Golgi proposed that the acid was formed within the surface invaginations, which he termed "secretory canaliculi". While these postulates were generally accepted, direct evidence was not obtained until methods became available for visualizing acid spaces in living cells nearly 90 years later.

Gastric parietal cells are located in the oxyntic [from the Greek *oxyno,* to make acid] glands found in the fundus and corpus of the stomach. The glands are easily identified in normal histological sections as shown in figure 2. Parietal cells are not normally found in the gastric antrum nor, except under pathological conditions such as Barrett's disease or duodenal gastric metaplasia, are they located in any other gastrointestinal organ. The oxyntic glands also contain peptic, or chief cells, mucus-secreting cells and a variety of neuro-endocrine cells. The parietal cells are identified easily on the basis of their relatively large size (20–25 μm diameter), their conical shape and the fact that they protrude from the wall of the gland, as suggested by their name (see figure 3). In the human stomach, parietal cells are most abundant in the neck region and middle portion of the oxyntic glands, while the peptic cells occupy most of the basal region (2,3). Neuro-endocrine cells are distributed sparsely throughout the glands and are small cells (ca. 10 μm diameter) which do not have access to the lumen of the gland.

Direct visualization of acid production by the parietal cell became possible with the development of isolated preparations of living gastric glands (4) and the use in this model of pH-sensitive metachromatic fluorescent dyes such as acridine orange (5). This dye is taken up by living cells and emits a green fluorescence. Because acridine orange is a weak base, it accumulates in acidic spaces, stacks and the fluorescence shifts to red. Use of this dye with living gastric glands provided dramatic proof that acid is secreted into the canaliculus of the parietal cell (figure 4 and 5). Moreover, it was shown that acid is secreted directly into the canaliculi only when the parietal cell is stimulated, invalidating the concept that acid is preformed and stored in the parietal cell prior to release during stimulation.

(text continues on p. 12)

FIG. 2. A hematoxylin and eosin stained section of gastric fundic epithelium, showing the surface mucus, the surface epithelial cells and the gastric glands containing both parietal and peptic cells. A gland is outlined by a rectangle.

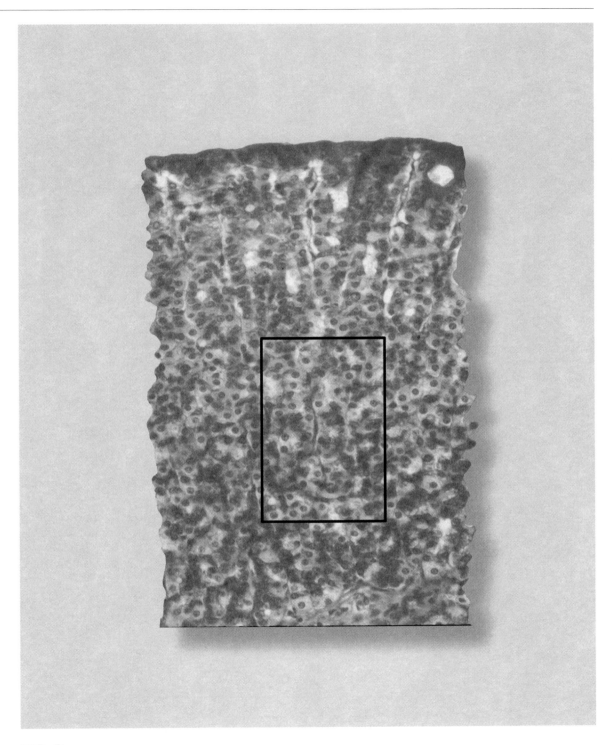

FIG. 2

FIG. 3 A scanning electron micrograph of an isolated gastric gland. The large parietal (i.e., peripheral) cells are seen bulging on the surface of this structure. The peptic cells are barely visible, hidden by the parietal cells.

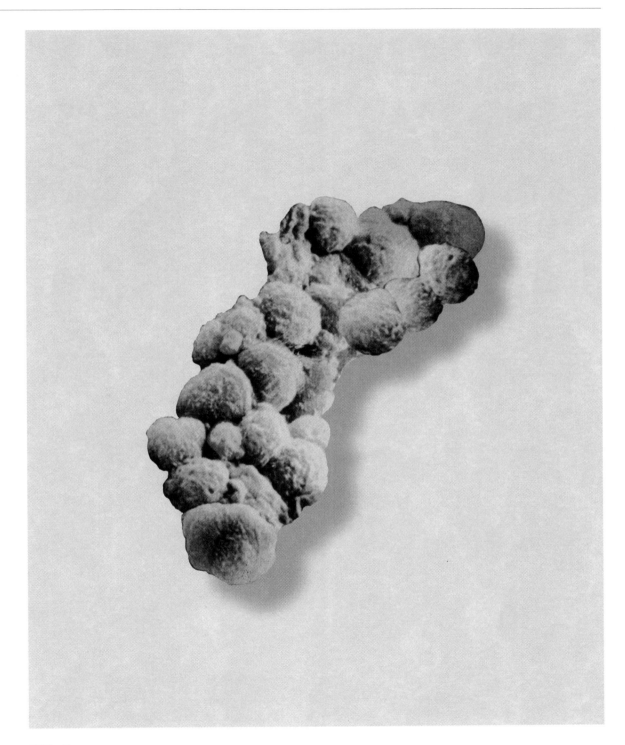

FIG. 3

FIG. 4 A fluorescent micrograph of a living gastric gland before stimulation, stained intravitally with the weak base dye acridine orange. The cytoplasm of the cells fluoresces green, and a more intense stain is seen in the lumen of the gland.

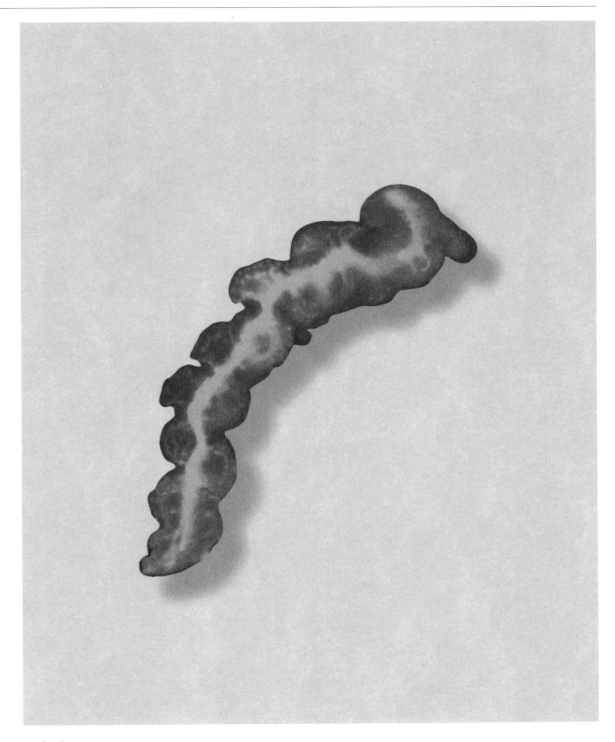

FIG. 4

FIG. 5 A fluorescent micrograph of a living gastric gland after stimulation of acid secretion, stained intravitally with the weak base acridine orange. This dye accumulates in acidic spaces, changing its fluorescence to red. The cytoplasm of the cells is still stained green, but the now acidic space of the intracellular canaliculi and the lumen of the gastric gland stains red. This observation shows that the site of acid secretion is the secretory canaliculus of the parietal cell.

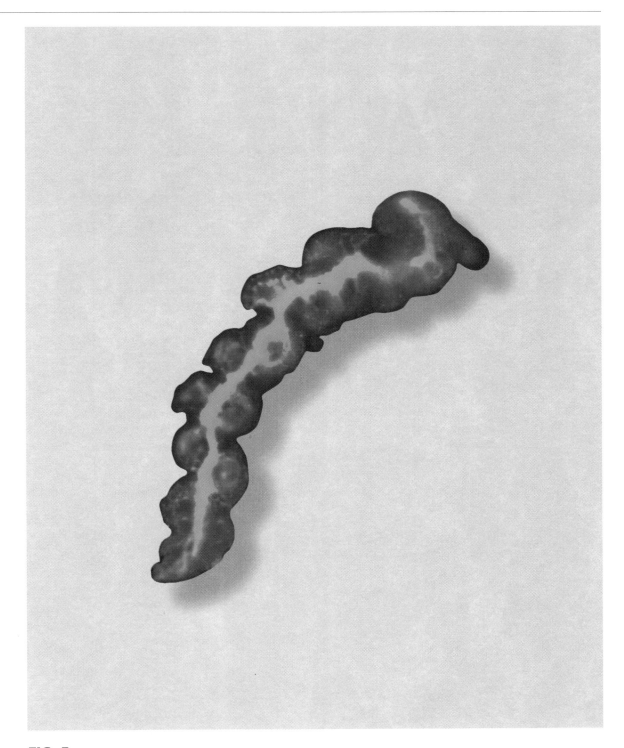

FIG. 5

■ Secretory Canaliculus

The ultrastructure of the parietal cell is distinctive. The cytoplasm is sparse and the cell contains numerous large mitochondria to provide the energy (ATP) for acid secretion. The most prominent feature of the cell is the presence of a secretory canaliculus which may be collapsed or expanded to nearly fill the cell, depending on the status of cell stimulation (6,7,8). Electron microscopy provided confirmation of the light microscopic observations of Golgi. In addition, electron microscopy revealed a feature of the parietal cell which could not be seen by Golgi, namely the presence of membrane-bounded structures, the cytoplasmic tubules. These tubular structures are numerous in parietal cells which contain only rudimentary canaliculi but are nearly absent upon full stimulation which results in a large expansion of the canalicular surface. After stimulation, the expanded canaliculi contain numerous microvilli containing actin filaments. Quantitative comparison of the membrane area contained in the tubules and secretory canaliculi under different conditions of secretory activity has led to the conclusion that expansion of the secretory canaliculi involves incorporation of the tubules into the canaliculus. The exact mechanism by which tubules are converted into canalicular membrane is not known. However it cannot be the same as the better-studied process of exocytosis. The functional consequence of this morphological change is to activate the parietal cell acid pump.

Following the initial identification of the gastric acid pump as an enzyme, the H^+,K^+-ATPase, it became possible to localize the pumps in the gastric mucosa by staining with specific antibodies (9). Such studies, illustrated in figures 7 and 8, demonstrated that the pumps are located both in cytoplasmic tubules and in the membrane of the secretory canaliculi, as was anticipated. In the resting cell the pump is in the tubule, in the stimulated cell in the canalicular membrane. The conclusion drawn from these observations is that during stimulation of the parietal cell, acid pumps are incorporated into the secretory canaliculi, along with the tubule membranes. Models depicting the distribution of pumps in the resting and stimulated states of the parietal cell are presented in figures 9 and 10. The pumps are not active when present in the cytoplasmic tubules but become active only when incorporated into the secretory membrane (5,10,11). Proton transport by the H^+,K^+-ATPase requires a supply of K^+ for the exchange process, as described below.

(text continues on p. 22)

FIG. 6. *A scanning electron micrograph of the surface of a single parietal cell, colored in shades of green, showing its characteristic conical shape. The apex of the cell faces the lumen of the gastric gland.*

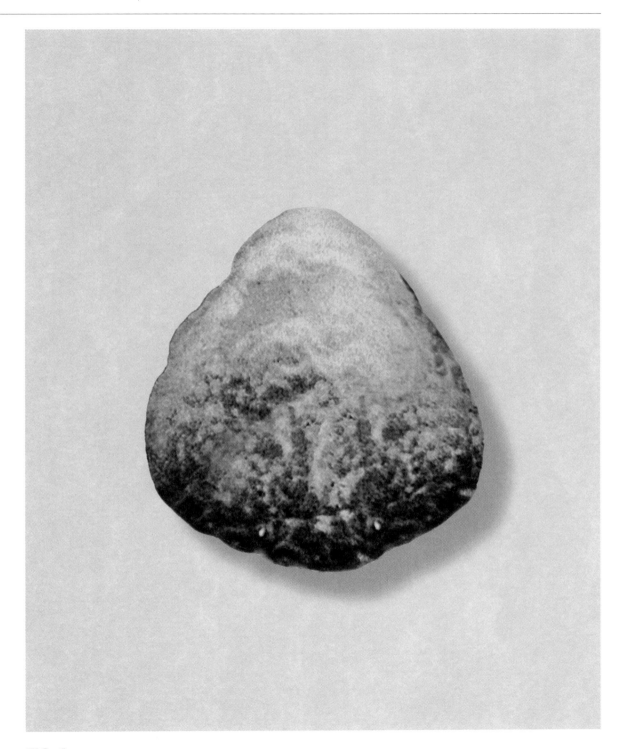

FIG. 6

FIG. 7. A transmission electron micrograph of a resting parietal cell, where the acid pump, the H^+,K^+-ATPase, has been stained with a specific antibody. The cytoplasm is colored green and the sites recognized by the antibody stained black. The pump is seen to be located in the cytoplasm in tubules cut in cross section. The cell contains many mitochondria and a collapsed secretory canaliculus.

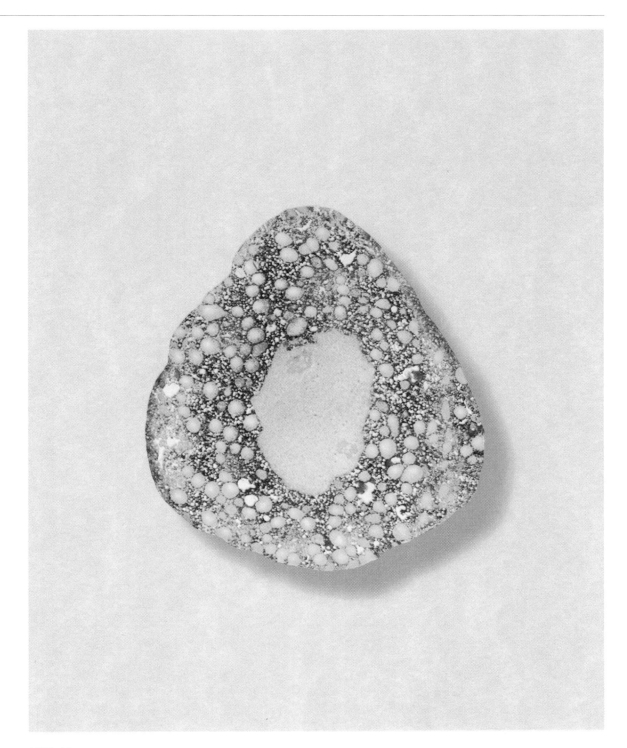

FIG. 7

FIG. 8. A transmission electron micrograph of a stimulated parietal cell, where the acid pump, the H+,K+-ATPase, has been stained with a specific antibody. The cytoplasm is colored green, the active secretory canaliculus is colored red, and the sites recognized by the antibody stained black. The pump is mostly in the microvilli lining the secretory canaliculus and has largely disappeared from the cytoplasm. The red colorization of the canalicular space correlates with the actual red acridine orange fluorescence seen at lower magnification in figure 5.

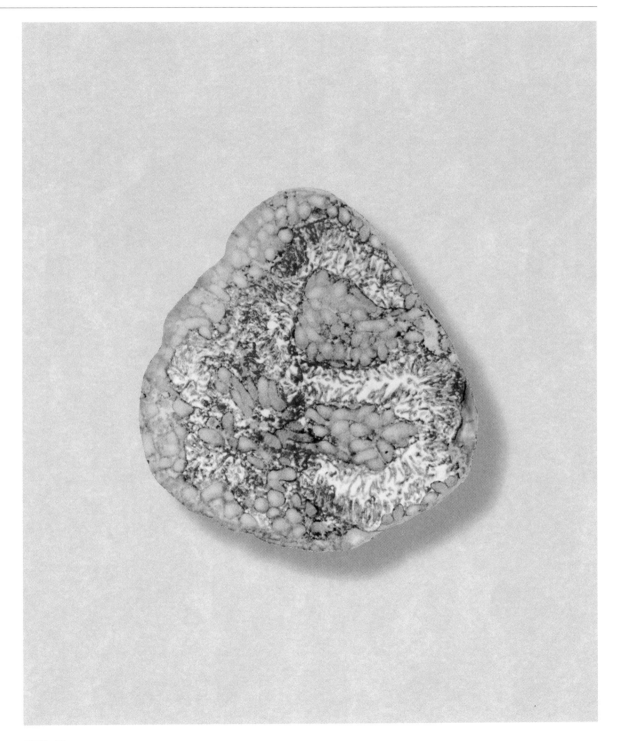

FIG. 8

FIG. 9. A conceptual model of an unstimulated parietal cell. This shows the relatively collapsed secretory canaliculus, and the inactive pumps mostly in small, tubular cytoplasmic structures. An active pump is colored red, the inactive pumps blue-gray. A single pump molecule is seen to be functional in the canaliculus of the parietal cell, producing a low flow of acid even in the absence of food stimulation in man. The seven membrane-spanning segment receptors at the base of the cell are inactive.

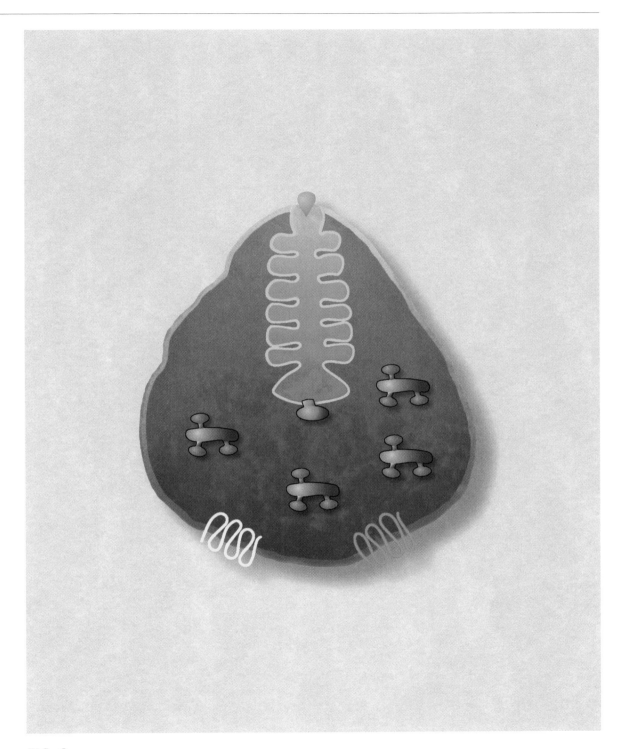

FIG. 9

FIG. 10. A conceptual model of a stimulated parietal cell. The pumps are now mostly in the membrane of the expanded secretory canaliculus. Associated with the pumps is a pathway allowing K+ and Cl⁻ to exit the cell. The K+ is pumped back into the cytoplasm by the ATPase in exchange for H+. This results in HCl and water extrusion into the canaliculus and out of the apex of the parietal cell into the lumen of the gastric gland. The cholinergic M_3 receptor activates the cell using intracellular calcium as a second messenger, whereas the histamine H_2 receptor activates the cell using cAMP as a second messenger. The function of the gastrin receptor of the parietal cell in acid secretion is not known.

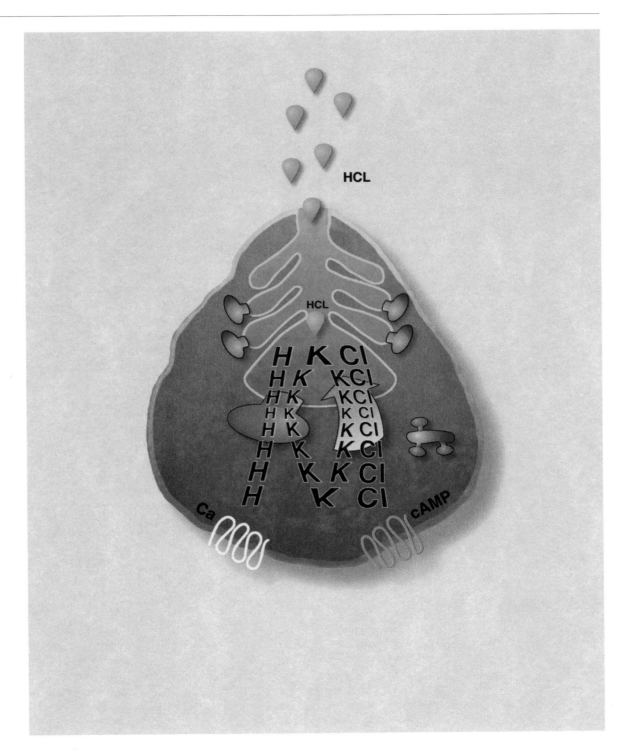

FIG. 10

Potassium ions are provided to the pump by a K^+,Cl^- transporter or by K^+ and Cl^- channels which are present in the membrane of the secretory canaliculi but absent or inactive in the membrane of the cytoplasmic tubules (10,12). It is likely that stimulation of the parietal cell results in an increased activity of the K^+,Cl^- transporters or channels in the canalicular membrane, in addition to the incorporation of acid pumps. The transport of K^+ and Cl^- into the canalicular lumen activates the ATPase-driven exchange process whereby the K^+ is recycled in exchange for H^+ and the Cl^- accumulates with the H^+, resulting in net secretion of isotonic HCl. The water accompanying the HCl is driven out of the cell by the efflux of KCl. The composition of the acidic fluid secreted by the parietal cell is therefore an isotonic mixture of largely HCl and some KCl.

The absence of functioning KCl transporters in the membrane of the cytoplasmic tubules prevents activity of the pumps when they are located in these structures. It is significant that, even with maximal stimulation of the parietal cell, not all of the acid pumps are incorporated into the canaliculi. There always is a fraction of the pumps which remain inactive in the cytoplasmic tubules. The distribution of acid pumps between the canaliculi and the tubules depends on the level of parietal cell stimulation. Under resting conditions less than 30% of the pumps are located in the canaliculi. Upon stimulation of the parietal cell there is a rapid transfer of pumps to the secretory membrane resulting in activation of 60–70% of the total pumps (10). This transfer occurs relatively quickly, being evident within 2 minutes and reaching a new steady state within 20 minutes (8,11,13). When the stimulus is withdrawn, the transfer is reversed, with acid pumps returning to their inactive state in the cytoplasmic tubules. The reversal process appears to be significantly slower than the activation process, requiring about 60 minutes for a complete return to the resting condition.

The incorporation of tubule membrane, together with acid pumps, into the secretory canaliculus and its subsequent recovery are now known to be part of a dynamic cycling process which occurs continuously in the parietal cell (10,11,13). The cytoskeleton of the cell (in particular the cytoskeletal proteins actin and ezrin (14)) is intimately involved in the morphological alteration between the resting and secreting parietal cell. The continuous cycling of pumps has important implications for the pharmacodynamics of covalent inhibitors such as omeprazole, as discussed in Section III.

GASTRIC ACID PUMP

The molecular mechanism of acid secretion by the parietal cell was controversial for decades. The discovery of adenosine triphosphate (ATP)-driven proton transport in gastric cell membranes (15) and of the enzyme responsible for this ion transport (16,17) led to the identification of the H^+,K^+-ATPase as the gastric acid pump. Over the past twenty years, substantial evidence has accumulated to show that the H^+,K^+-ATPase is the final molecular step in acid secretion.

■ Transport by the H^+,K^+-ATPase, the Gastric Acid Pump

The H^+,K^+-ATPase is a membrane-embedded protein which exchanges protons for potassium. As a function of the hydrolysis of ATP, hydrogen ions pass from the cytoplasmic side of the pump, through the membrane domain, and are released to the outside or extracytosolic surface of the enzyme. In exchange for this outward movement of hydrogen ions there is an inward movement of potassium ions. Since the transport of both hydrogen and potassium ions is against their electrochemical gradient, the overall process requires a net expenditure of energy. Indeed, the gastric secretion of hydrogen ions generates a concentration gradient for H^+ in excess of four million, from a cytoplasmic pH of 7.3 to a luminal pH of 0.8. This makes gastric acid secretion one of the most efficient transport processes known in biology and severely restricts the types of chemical reactions which could supply sufficient energy to drive the transport. The gastric acid pump utilizes the chemical energy contained in the terminal phosphate bond of ATP to achieve this remarkable pH gradient.

Considerable effort over the last two decades led to a description of the enzymatic and transport reactions of the H^+,K^+-ATPase (18). These reactions, referred to as the catalytic cycle, involve a change in the conformation of the enzyme such that the sites for ion binding change their affinity and sidedness (figure 11). The conformational change is brought about by phosphorylation and dephosphorylation of the protein during hydrolysis of ATP. One conformation of the protein, designated E_1, binds hydrogen (or hydronium) ions with a high affinity at the cytoplasmic surface and becomes phosphorylated by ATP. Upon phosphorylation the hydrogen ion is entrapped, or occluded, within the membrane domain of the enzyme. This form spontaneously converts to the second conformation of the protein, the E_2 conformation, while remaining phosphorylated. The E_2 form has a low-affinity binding site for hydrogen ion exposed to the extracytoplasmic surface and releases the hydrogen ion to the outside. After H^+ is released, K^+ can bind to the outside surface with high affinity. Phosphate is released from the enzyme as K^+ becomes occluded in the membrane domain. Release of K^+ to the cytoplasmic side occurs as the protein spontaneously converts back to the E_1 conformation, completing the transport cycle. The overall result of this catalytic cycle is the hydrolysis of ATP accompanied by an equal exchange of hydrogen for potassium ions. The obligatory exchange of potassium accounts for the inactivity of the acid pumps when they are located in the cytoplasmic tubules. The tubule membranes are impermeable to potassium, and therefore lack the K^+ on their luminal surface which is necessary for completion of the pump cycle. The ion transported outward by the ATPase is probably the hydrated proton, the hydronium ion, H_3O^+ (19). The mechanism of ion transport by this pump is therefore very similar to the mechanism of transport of Na^+ and K^+ by the ubiquitous sodium pump (20). Since pumping is dependent on shape changes of the protein, this biological pump can be thought of as a chemo-mechanical pump, the conversion of scalar chemical energy into vectorial ion transport being achieved by changes in protein conformation.

(text continues on p. 26)

FIG. 11. The catalytic cycle of the H^+,K^+-ATPase. The pump protein binds H^+ as the hydrated form, the hydronium ion, H_3O^+. The protein is then energized by ATP, to form the phosphorylated form, E_1-P, that allows transport of the ion from cytoplasm into lumen. This ion translocation occurs as the pump changes conformation from the E_1-P.H_3O^+ form to the E_2-P.H_3O^+ form through the occluded E.P[H_3O^+] form. In this E_2 form, the pump releases H_3O^+ and then binds K^+ from the luminal side and transports it back to the cytoplasmic side via the E.[K^+] occluded form as phosphate is released from the protein. The E_1.K^+ form releases the K^+ and rebinds the hydronium ion to allow the cycle to start again.

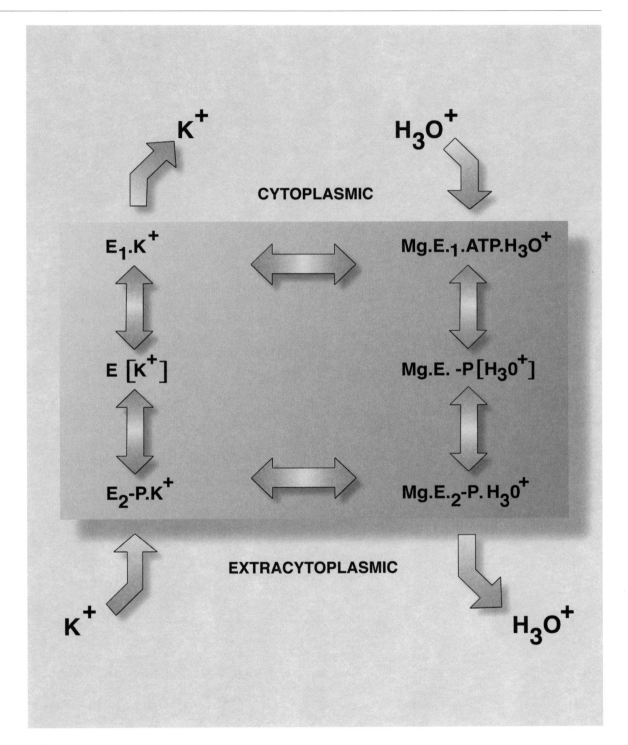

FIG. 11

■ Structure of the H+,K+-ATPase

The H[+],K[+]-ATPase was initially identified and isolated as a membrane-embedded protein in the 1970's. Analysis of the membranes containing the K[+]-dependent ATPase indicated that it consisted of a single polypeptide having a molecular mass of about 100,000 (21). The antibodies employed to localize the H[+],K[+]-ATPase were generated against this polypeptide (9). More recent studies have revealed that the H[+],K[+]-ATPase actually consists of two dissimilar subunits (22). The larger of the two, consisting of a chain of 1033 or 1034 amino acids, is the polypeptide originally identified and is referred to as the α subunit, or as the catalytic subunit (23). The latter term is in recognition of the fact that this subunit contains the functional sites of the enzyme. The second subunit, the β subunit, is much smaller, consisting of approximately 290 amino acids (24). The amino acid sequences are shown in figure 12. The two subunits are found to associate in a one to one ratio and this α,β complex is believed to represent a functional pump unit.

Both subunits of the H[+],K[+]-ATPase traverse the lipid bilayer of the membrane in which the pump is embedded (see figure 13). The large subunit threads in and out of the bilayer several times (25), with most of its amino acids found in large cytoplasmic loops between membrane-spanning segments. The membrane segments are connected by extracytoplasmic loops. The cytoplasmic loops contain sites for ATP binding and phosphorylation (26). The smaller β subunit has a single membrane-spanning segment with most of its amino acids found in the extracytoplasmic space (24). The extracytoplasmic domain of the β subunit is heavily glycosylated and contains three internal disulfide bridges. Although it is not thought to be directly involved in the transport reactions of the H[+],K[+]-ATPase, the β subunit is essential for directing newly synthesized pumps to the cytoplasmic tubules of the parietal cell and for stabilizing the enzymically active conformation of the α subunit. The three disulfide bridges of the β subunit are critical for maintaining a functional conformation of the α subunit (27).

(text continues on p. 30)

FIG. 12. The linear amino acid sequence of the two subunits of the H+,K+-ATPase. The larger α or catalytic subunit consists of 1033 amino acids in the hog, expressed as single letter codes. Highlighted are the transmembrane segments and their connecting extracytoplasmic loops as well as the cysteines, some of which are potential target amino acids for omeprazole. The smaller β subunit in the hog consists of 291 amino acids, mostly in the extracytoplasmic space, with one membrane-spanning segment. The cysteines in this space are disulfide-linked. There are also six potential N-linked glycosylation sites (NXT or NXS).

```
   1   MGKAENYELY QVELGPGPSP DMAAKMSKKK AGRGGGKRKE KLENMKKEME INDHQLSVAE

  61   LEQKYQTSAT KGLSASLAAE LLLRDGPMAL RPPRGTPEYV KFARQLAGGLQCLMWVAAAI      1

 121   CLIAFAIQAS EGDLTTDDNL YLALALLAVV VVTGCFGYYQ EFKSTNIIAS FKNLVPQQAT      2

 181   VIRDGDKFQI NADQLVVGDL VEMKGGDRVP ADIRILQAQG RKVDNSSLTG ESEPQTRSPE

 241   CTHESPLETR NIAFFSTMCL EGTAQGLVVN TGDRTIIGRI ASLASGVENE KTPIAIEIEH

 301   FVDIIAGLAI LFGATFFIVA MCIGYTFLRA MVFFMAIVVA YVPEGLLATV TVCLSLTAKR      3 4

 361   LASKNCVVKNLEAVETLGST SVICSDKTGT LTQNRMTVSH LWFDNHIHSA DTTEDQSGQT

 421   FDQSSETWRA LCRVLTLCNR AAFKSGQDAV PVPKRIVIGD ASETALLKFS ELTLGNAMGY

 481   RERFPKVCEI PFNSTNKFQL SIHTLEDPRD PRHVLVMKGA PERVLERCSS ILIKGQELPL

 541   DEQWREAFQT AYLSLGGLGE RVLGFCQLYL SEKDYPPGYA FDVEAMNFPT SGLSFAGLVS

 601   MIDPPRATVP DAVLKCRTAG IRVIMVTGDH PITAKAIAAS VGIISEGSET VEDAARLRV

 661   PVDQVNRKDA RACVINGMQL KDMDPSELVE ALRTHPEMVF ARTSPQQKLV IVESCQLGA

 721   IVAVTGDGVN DSPALKKADI GVAMGIAGSD AAKNAADMIL LDDNFASIVT GVEQGRLIFD

 781   NLKKSIAYTL TKNIPELTPY LIYITVSVPL PLGCITILFI ELCTDIFPSV SLAYEKAESD      5 6

 841   IMHLRPRNPK RDRLVNEPLA AYSYFQIGAI QSFAGFTDYF TAMAQEGWFP LLCVGLRPQW      7

 901   ENHHLQDLQD SYGQEWTFGQ RLYQQYTCYT VFFISIEMCQ IADVLIRKTR RLSAFQQGFF      8

 961   RNRILVIAIV FQVCIGCFLC YCPGMPNIFN FMPIRFQWWL VPMPFGLLIF VYDEIRKLGV      9 10

1021   RCCPGSWWDQ ELYY
```

```
   1   MAALQEKKSCSQRMEEFQRYCWNPDTGQML GRTLSRWVWI SLYYVAFYVV MSGIFALCIY

  61   VLMRTIDPYT PDYQDQLKSP GVTLRPDVYG EKGLDISYNV SDSTTWAGLA HTLHRFLAGY

 121   SPAAQEGSIN CTSEKYFFQE SFLAPNHTKF SCKFTADMLQ NCSGRPDPTF GFAEGKPCFI

 181   IKMNRIVKFL PGNSTAPRVD CAFLDQPRDG PPLQVEYFPA NGTYSLHYFP YYGKKAQPHY

 241   SNPLVAAKLL NVPRNRDVVI VCKILAEHVS FDNPHDPYEG KVEFKLKIQK
```

FIG. 12

FIG. 13. The two dimensional arrangement of the large catalytic subunit of the gastric pump to illustrate in some more detail the membrane and extra-cytoplasmic domain. There are certainly eight and perhaps ten membrane-spanning segments, with their interconnecting loops on the cytoplasmic and extracytoplasmic face. The amino acids are presented as single letter codes. The β subunit is shown folded around the TM7/TM8 connecting loop of the α subunit, with three disulfide bridges. The most hydrophilic amino acids in the membrane-spanning domain of the α subunit are highlighted.

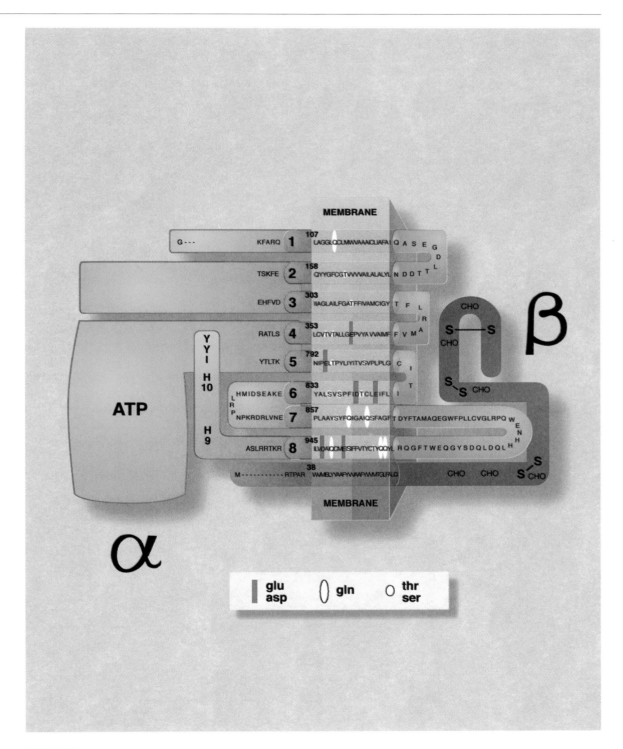

FIG. 13

The tertiary structure of the H^+,K^+-ATPase is not known, although knowledge of this is essential to understand how the enzyme performs its transport functions. Based on the known secondary structure and available information on functional domains, it is possible to envisage a reasonable model for the structure of the membrane-spanning domain of the α subunit of the H^+,K^+-ATPase and to attempt an explanation for the mechanism of action of proton pump inhibitors. Such a model is illustrated in figures 14, 15 and 16. The catalytic subunit has a large cytoplasmic domain; almost 80% of the amino acid residues are found in the cytoplasmic loops. In contrast, the extracytoplasmic domain contains only about 75 out of over 1000 amino acid residues and must be relatively small. The membrane-spanning domain consists of at least eight, and probably ten (25), helical segments of about 20 amino acids each, which are closely associated with each other to form a compact bundle. This is connected to the cytoplasmic domain by a stalk, as deduced from images of the Ca^{2+} ATPase of sarcoplasmic reticulum (32).

Since the transported ions pass through the membrane domain, the membrane-spanning segments must form the boundary of the ion transport pathway across the membrane. Charged or other hydrophilic amino acid residues, such as aspartic and glutamic acid, within the membrane domain would be most likely to participate in transport of cations such as H^+ or K^+. The carbonyl moiety of the peptide bonds may also participate, making intuitive predictions somewhat difficult, however. Nevertheless, analysis of the distribution of charged or hydrophilic residues suggests that many of the membrane-spanning segments contained in the carboxy terminus one third of the protein, especially segments 5 to 8, may contain most of the ion transport pathway. Whatever the exact arrangement of the transmembrane segments, the binding of ATP to, and phosphorylation/dephosphorylation of, the cytoplasmic domain must induce a conformational rearrangement in the protein. The pumping action of the protein depends on the conformational changes that determine the sidedness and affinity of the ion-binding sites. These conformational changes extrude H^+ across the membrane domain and reabsorb K^+ across the same domain.

(text continues on p. 36)

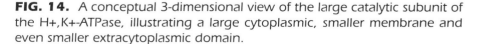

FIG. 14. *A conceptual 3-dimensional view of the large catalytic subunit of the H+,K+-ATPase, illustrating a large cytoplasmic, smaller membrane and even smaller extracytoplasmic domain.*

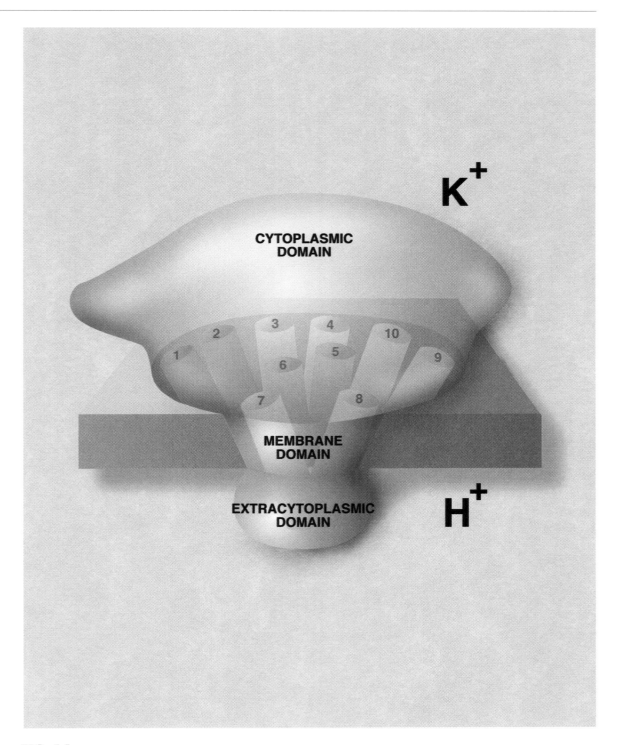

FIG. 14

FIG. 15. A cutaway of figure 14, to illustrate the possible 3-dimensional arrangement of the membrane-spanning segments and the extracytoplasmic loops.

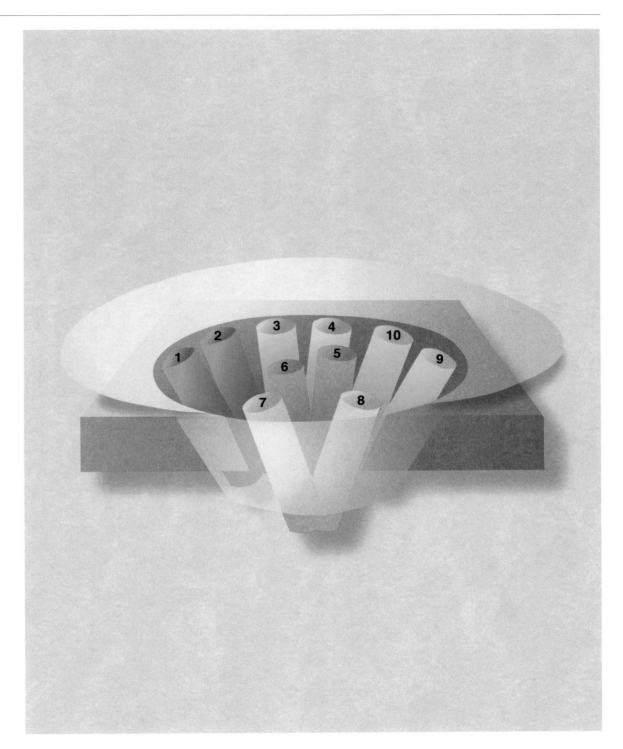

FIG. 15

FIG. 16. The membrane-spanning segments of the catalytic subunit, illustrating the potential ion pathway across the membrane domain of the pump. The ion pathway includes membrane segments 5,6 and 7,8 cytosolic H^+ passing out through this sector and luminal K^+ passing into the cell through this region. Inhibition of the pump from the extracytoplasmic surface should occur if a drug binds to the extracytoplasmic surface, particularly in the TM5/TM6 region.

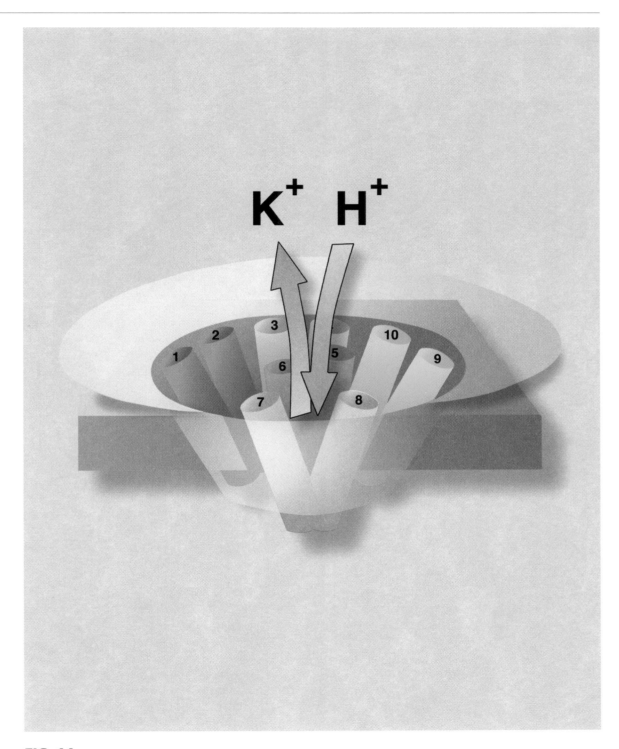

FIG. 16

BIOLOGY OF THE ACID PUMP

In the parietal cell the H^+,K^+-ATPase exists in two states, active and inactive, as discussed above. In both states the enzyme consists of α,β heterodimers and possesses the capability of proton transport provided K^+ is supplied to its luminal surface (10). The conversion from inactive to active state is not thought to involve any modification of the pump itself but depends on an association with a K^+,Cl^- transporter to provide K^+ at the extracytoplasmic exchange site. This association occurs only when the pump is located in the secretory canaliculus, and not when it is in the cytoplasmic tubules. Thus, the canaliculus is the only site of acid formation in the parietal cell but not the only location of acid pumps.

The translocation of pumps from the tubules into the canaliculus and their retrieval is a continuous process that continues even in the absence of overt stimulation in most species. For the unstimulated parietal cell, about 4% of the pumps cycle through the canalicular membrane every hour (11). Thus, without stimulation, all of the pumps would be expected to cycle through the active state about once every 24 hours.

Stimulation of the parietal cell by activation of cellular receptors leads to an increase in the rate of insertion of pumps into the secretory canaliculus and thus to an increase in the number of active acid pumps present in the canaliculus. Short term stimulation does not, however, result in any increase in the total number of pumps, active plus inactive, in the parietal cell (10). During sustained stimulation the pumps continue to cycle into and out of the canaliculus so as to maintain a distribution of pumps between the active and inactive membranes which is dependent on the intensity of the stimulus. With cessation of the stimulus the rate of pump insertion slows allowing the retrieval process to reduce the number of active pumps in the secretory canaliculus and thus reduce the rate of acid secretion.

The total number of acid pumps in the parietal cell appears to be relatively constant. This finding does not mean that the H^+,K^+-ATPase protein does not turn over. As with most cellular proteins, the H^+,K^+-ATPase undergoes a continuous process of degradation and synthesis (figure 17). The pump protein half life has been mea-

FIG. 17. The biosynthesis and catabolism of the gastric H+,K+-ATPase. Shown is the synthesis of the α and β subunits of the pump, with initial assembly in the endoplasmic reticulum. This is followed by processing in the Golgi, especially of the β subunit. From the late Golgi, the tubules are formed that contain the mature pump. These tubules cycle in and out of the active secretory canaliculus, where a K+,Cl- pathway is activated. Some of the pump present in the secretory canaliculus, rather than in the tubules, is taken up into endosomes and thence into secondary lysosomes and is catabolized. The half life of the pump is about 50 hrs in rats.

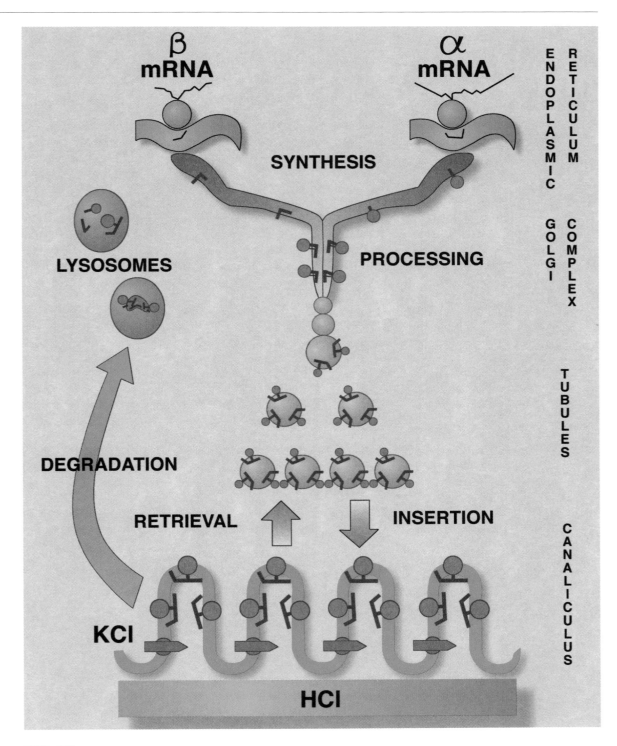

FIG. 17

sured directly in the rat and is about 50 hours (28). Degradation of the pump protein depends on recognition of older or functioning molecules. It has been found that ranitidine, an H_2 receptor antagonist which results in withdrawal of the pump from the active membrane, doubles the half life of the pump. Omeprazole is without effect on the half life (29). Thus it may be that the half life of the pump is use dependent, pump molecules being broken down mainly when stimulated and remaining relatively stable when unstimulated. This recognition of the secreting rather than the resting pump facilitates on the average degradation of older protein molecules.

The biosynthesis of acid pumps occurs on the membranes of the endoplasmic reticulum. It is likely that synthesis of both α and β subunits from their respective mRNA's occurs virtually simultaneously, since the proteins associate early in the processing pathway and an excess of one subunit over the other has not been found. The mature α subunit is not glycosylated, but the β subunit is glycosylated in the endoplasmic reticulum. The carbohydrates of this subunit are processed further in the Golgi apparatus to their mature form. The glycosylation is presumably necessary for targeting the mature complex to the cytoplasmic tubules. From the trans Golgi the mature pump vesicles bud off to form the cytoplasmic tubules containing H^+,K^+-ATPase in the inactive state.

The rate of pump synthesis is regulated, at least in part, at the level of gene expression. Nucleotide sequences preceding the sequence coding for the pump subunits are recognized by cellular transcription factors such as specific proteins or small molecules, e.g., cyclic AMP or calcium. These bind to the DNA upstream to the transcription initiation site and stimulate the transcription of mRNA coding for the pump protein.

It has been shown that elevated mucosal histamine transiently stimulates pump mRNA transcription and that this stimulation is blocked by H_2 receptor antagonists (30). On the other hand in rabbits, long-term inhibition of acid secretion by H_2 receptor antagonists elevates the level of the H^+,K^+-ATPase: long term inhibition of acid secretion by omeprazole decreases the level of the H^+,K^+-ATPase (31). These findings may explain why acid rebound often occurs after the use of H_2 receptor antagonists and generally is not observed after omeprazole administration. The two classes of acid secretory inhibitors also have distinct effects on parietal cell morphology; the H_2 receptor antagonists induce a resting state, whereas the pump inhibitors appear to exaggerate a stimulated morphology (30). Using current therapy, however, these morphological effects are transient.

REFERENCES

1. Golgi, C.: Sur la fine organisation des glandes peptiques des mammiferes. Arch. Ital. Biol. 19, 448, 1893.

2. Helander, H. F.: The cells of the gastric mucosa. Internat. Rev. Cytol. 70, 217, 1981.

3. Ito, S.: Functional gastric morphology. In, Johnson, L. R. (ed), Physiology of the Gastrointestinal Tract. Vol 1, 2nd edition, New York, Raven Press, p. 817, 1987.

4. Berglindh, T., Helander, H. F., and Obrink, K. J.: Effects of secretagogues on oxygen consumption, aminopyrine accumulation and morphology in isolated gastric glands. Acta Physiol. Scand. 97, 401, 1976.

5. Dibona, D. R., Ito, S., Berglindh, T., and Sachs, G.: Cellular site of gastric acid secretion. Proc. Natl. Acad. Sci. USA 76, 6689, 1979.

6. Helander, H. F., and Hirschowitz, B.I.: Quantitative ultrastructural studies on gastric parietal cells. Gastroenterology 63, 951, 1972.

7. Ito S., and Schofield, G.C.: Studies on the depletion and accumulation of microvilli and changes in the tubulovesicular compartment of mouse parietal cells in relation to gastric acid secretion. J. Cell Biol. 63, 364, 1974.

8. Gibert, A. J., and Hersey, S.J.: Morphometric analysis of parietal cell membrane transformations in isolated gastric glands. J. Membrane Biol. 67, 113, 1982.

9. Smolka, A., Helander, H. F., and Sachs, G.: Monoclonal antibodies against gastric H^+,K^+ ATPase. Am. J. Physiol. 245, G589, 1983

10. Hersey, S. J., Perez, A., Matheravidathu, S., and Sachs, G.: Gastric H^+K^+-ATPase in situ, evidence for compartmentalization. Am. J. Physiol. 257, G539, 1989.

11. Scott, D. R., Helander, H. F., Hersey, S. J., and Sachs, G.: The site of acid secretion in the mammalian parietal cell. Biochim. Biophys. Acta 1146, 73, 1993.

12. Wolosin, J. M., and Forte, J.G.: Stimulation of oxyntic cells triggers K^+ and Cl– conductances in apical H^+K^+-ATPase membrane. Am. J. Physiol. 246, C537– , 1984.

13. Forte, T. M., Machen, T. E., and Forte, J.G.: Ultrastructural changes in oxyntic cells associated with secretory function. A membrane recycling hypothesis. Gastroenterology 73, 941, 1977.

14. Yao, X., Thibodeau, A., and Forte, J.G.: Ezrin-calpain I interactions in gastric parietal cells. Am. J. Physiol. 265, C36, 1993.

15. Lee, J., Simpson, G., and Scholes, P.: An ATPase from dog gastric mucosa, changes of outer pH in suspensions of dog membrane vesicles accompanying ATP hydrolysis. Biochem. Biophys. Res. Commun. 60, 825, 1974.

16. Ganser, A. L. and Forte, J. G.: K^+-stimulated ATPase in purified microsomes of bullfrog oxyntic cells. Biochim. Biophys. Acta 307, 169, 1973.

17. Sachs, G., Chang, H. H., Rabon E., Schackman, R., Lewin, M., and Saccomani, G.: A non-electrogenic H^+ pump in plasma membranes of hog stomach. J. Biol. Chem. 251, 7690, 1976.

18. Sachs, G.: The gastric H,K ATPase, regulation and structure/function of the acid pump of the stomach, in Physiology of the gastrointestinal tract, Johnson LR ed, p1119 Raven Press, 1994.

19. Polvani, C., Sachs, G., and Blostein, R.: Sodium ions as substitutes for protons in the gastric H^+K^+-ATPase. J. Biol. Chem. 264, 17854, 1989.

20. Glynn, I. M. and Karlish, S. J.: Occluded ions in active transport. Ann. Rev. Biochem. 59, 171, 1990.

21. Saccomani, G., Stewart, H. B., Shaw, D., Lewin, M., and Sachs, G.: Characterization of gastric mucosal membranes. IX. Fractionation and purification of K^+-ATPase containing vesicles by zonal centrifugation and free-flow electrophoresis. Biochim. Biophys. Acta 465, 311, 1977.

22. Hall, K., Perez, G., Anderson, D., Gutierrez, C., Munson, K. B., Hersey, S. J., Kaplan, J. H., and Sachs, G.: Location of carbohydrates present in the H^+K^+-ATPase vesicles isolated from hog gastric mucosa. Biochemistry 29, 701, 1990.

23. Shull, G. E., and Lingrel, J. B.: Molecular cloning of the rat stomach H^+K^+-ATPase. J. Biol. Chem. 261, 16788, 1986.

24. Reuben, M. A., Lasater, L. S., and Sachs, G.: Characterization of a beta subunit of the gastric H^+K^+-ATPase. Proc. Natl. Acad. Sci. USA 87, 6767, 1990.

25. Besancon, M., Shin, J. M., Mercier, F., Munson, K., Miller, M., Hersey, S. J. and Sachs, G.: Membrane topology and omeprazole labelling of the gastric H^+K^+-ATPase. Biochemistry 32, 2345, 1993.

26. Walderhaug, M. O., Post, R. L., Saccomani, G., Leonard, R. T., and Briskin, D.P.: Structural relatedness of three ion-transport adenosine triphosphatases around their active sites of phosphorylation. J. Biol. Chem. 260, 3852, 1985.

27. Shin, J. M. S., Besancon, M., Simon, A., and Sachs, G.: The site of pantoprazole in the gastric H^+K^+-ATPase. Biochim. Biophys. Acta 1148, 223, 1993.

28. Gedda, K., Scott, D., Besancon, M., and Sachs,G.: The half life of the H,K ATPase of gastric mucosa. Gastroenterology 106, A79, 1994.(Abstract)

29. Gedda, K., Scott, D., Besancon, M., and Sachs,G.: The effect of omeprazole and ranitidine on the half life of the gastric ATPase. Gastroenterology, in press, 1995.

30. Tari, A., Yamamoto, G., Sumii, K., Sumii, M., Takehara, Y., Harumna, K., Kajiyama, G., Wu, V., Sachs, G., and Walsh, J.: The role of histamine-2 receptor in the expression of rat gastric H^+K^+-ATPase. Am. J. Physiol. 265, G752 1993

31. Scott, D. R., Besancon, M., Helander H.F. and Sachs, G.: Effects of antisecretory agents on parietal cell structure and H+,K+-ATPase levels in rabbit gastric mucosa in vivo. Amer J Dig Dis and Sci 39, 2118, 1994

32. Toyoshima, C., Sasabe, H., and Stokes, D. L.: Three-dimensional cryo-electron microscopy of the calcium ion pump in the sarcoplasmic reticulum membrane. Nature 362, 467, 1993.

Regulation of
Acid Secretion

OVERVIEW

Production of gastric acid requires stimulation of the parietal cell. Both central and peripheral mechanisms are involved in activating cellular receptors on the gastric parietal cell.

The central nervous system integrates sensory information arising from the special senses, central chemoreceptors, and visceral sensory receptors. Efferent stimulatory impulses are transmitted through the vagus nerve to the peripheral neurons of the enteric nervous system.

The enteric nervous system integrates the vagal input with peripheral sensory information and regulates the release of transmitter substances which activate the parietal cell. The most important transmitter substances are acetylcholine, released from enteric nerve fibers, and histamine, released from enterochromaffin-like (ECL) cells. The stimulation of the ECL cell to release histamine is the major regulatory pathway for stimulation of acid secretion by the parietal cell.

The major peripheral mechanism for regulating gastric acid secretion is the plasma gastrin level. It is elevated by food in the antrum (probably mainly aromatic amino acids), and the level is decreased by inhibition of gastrin secretion by low (pH ≤ 3) intragastric pH. This acidity-dependent suppression of gastrin release at pH below 3 represents the most important mechanism for preventing excessive acid secretion. An intragastric pH level above 3 in the presence of food in the stomach can lead to hypergastrinemia.

The release of histamine by the enterochromaffin-like cells plays a central role in peripheral regulation of acid secretion. Histamine is released from the ECL cells by gastrin and acetylcholine.

The primary mechanism leading to the release of histamine from the ECL cell is through the hormone gastrin. Secretion of gastrin by the G-cell of the gastric antrum is stimulated by enteric nerve fibers and by the presence of food in the stomach. Gastrin travels through the circulation to the fundic mucosa, where it acts on the ECL cells at a CCK-B subtype peptide receptor to initiate histamine release.

Histamine release from the ECL cell also is stimulated by acetylcholine, released from enteric nerve fibers, acting at perhaps a pharmacological M_1 subtype muscarinic receptor. The histamine released from the ECL cell by the neural and hormonal mechanisms acts as a paracrine agent to stimulate nearby parietal cells.

The transmitters which act directly on the parietal cell bind to its specific receptors, the histamine H_2 receptor and the acetylcholine M_3 receptor. The hormone gastrin binds to a CCK-B receptor on the parietal cell. Activation of these receptors elevates the level of intracellular second messengers, cyclic AMP, and intracellular calcium, respectively, which in turn activate the steps leading to acid secretion by the parietal cell.

The figures illustrating regulation of acid secretion are figures 18 through 24.

MECHANISMS OF STIMULATION

In the total absence of stimuli parietal cells do not secrete acid. In man there is a continuous low level of basal acid production reflecting the chronic presence of low levels of stimulation. Digestive levels of acid production occur only upon activation of stimulatory pathways. There are several pathways which activate the parietal cell, involving the central nervous system, the vagus nerve, the enteric nervous system, and several endocrine cells of the gastric mucosa.

Central Stimulation

The sight, smell, taste or thought of food can initiate stimulatory responses within the central nervous system. The central initiation of acid secretion, often referred to as the `cephalic phase' of secretion, represents but one element in an integrated system of control mechanisms which allow higher organisms to regulate their feeding behavior, their gastrointestinal functions, and ultimately their nutritional homeostasis.

The central nervous system (CNS) initiates acid secretion via the vagus nerve (1,2,3). Efferent fibers of the vagus arising from the dorsomotor nucleus of the vagus (DMNV) within the medulla convey stimulatory signals to the stomach. The nuclei of the medulla, primarily the DMNV, serve as true regulatory centers in that they integrate cognitive, sensory, and nutritional inputs to modulate the vagal outflow. While the special sensory inputs, sight, smell and taste, are most commonly associated with the central regulation of acid secretion, other, less obvious, sensory inputs are involved. Hypoglycemia, detected by glucose sensors of the hypothalamus and relayed to DMNV, is one of the most potent factors in the central stimulation of acid secretion (2). The observation that ninety-seven percent of the vagal fibers (4) are afferent sensory fibers indicates that the medullary centers are critically involved in integrating visceral sensory information. Visceral sensory signals arise from mechanoreceptors detecting distention of the stomach and intestine and from chemoreceptors detecting specific components of the luminal contents. Central integration serves to adjust acid secretion to meet the requirements of peripheral conditions while avoiding excessive acid production.

Peripheral Stimulation

The efferent vagal fibers do not synapse directly with epithelial cells of the gastric mucosa but terminate on ganglion cells (5) of the enteric nervous system (ENS). The ENS is a dense nerve network with analogy to the CNS in having glial cells and a blood-ganglion barrier. The ENS contains virtually as many neurons as the spinal cord and is capable of initiating basic gastric functions such as secretion and motility in the absence of any extrinsic input. The primary role of the vagal input is to modulate the intrinsic activity of the ENS (5).

Efferent vagal fibers synapse with only about one out of 5000 enteric neurons, consistent with a modulatory role (5). The efferent vagal synapses are primarily cholinergi-nicotinic in nature, consistent with other parasympathetic preganglionic synapses. Within the ENS, interneuronal synapses also are cholinergic but some are muscarinic, since they are inhibited by atropine. In addition, enteric neurons contain a variety of biogenic amines and peptide neurotransmitters. These substances are postulated to play a role in regulating motility and gastric secretion. However, specific functions for these individual substances have not been defined (6).

The gastric ENS contains primary sensory fibers which detect distention, i.e., mechanoreceptors, and the constituents of the gastric juice, i.e., chemoreceptors. This sensory information is relayed through the ENS to afferent vagal fibers and thence to the central regulatory centers. The mechanochemical sensory information is integrated also within the ENS to regulate local reflex mechanisms and the release of the hormone gastrin and the paracrine agent histamine (5).

Neuronal activation of acid secretion involves three primary pathways: direct stimulation by enteric nerve fibers, release of histamine from ECL cells, and release of gastrin from G-cells of the gastric antrum. Inhibition of acid secretion probably involves release of somatostatin from the D cell of gastric fundus and antrum. This general mechanism of stimulation is illustrated in figure 18.

A small percentage of enteric neurons send projections to the mucosal layer of the stomach. These fibers do not form traditional synapses with individual epithelial cells. Instead, these fibers exhibit periodic swellings or varicosities which contain neurotransmitter storage granules and are presumed to be the site for transmitter release. The neurotransmitter, primarily acetylcholine, is released into the interstitial space, where it diffuses to nearby epithelial cells. Within the fundus and body of the stomach, acetylcholine can diffuse directly to the parietal cells, where it binds to a muscarinic M_3 type receptor (7,8). Binding to this receptor activates the parietal cell to secrete acid. It should be noted that the direct stimulation of the parietal cell by acetylcholine alone does not result in as high a rate of acid secretion as is observed with histamine alone.

A second pathway for neural activation of acid secretion is mostly indirect. This occurs by release of the hormone gastrin from the G-cell with neural stimulation. Gastrin also serves as the primary endocrine mediator of acid secretion induced by the presence of food in the stomach. This hormonal pathway acts primarily through the ECL cell to release histamine, which in turn activates gastric parietal cells.

The antral mucosa contains endocrine cells, the G-cells, which synthesize and secrete the peptide hormone gastrin. Gastrin secretion is stimulated by acetylcholine released from the enteric nerve fibers (2) and by cholinergic agonists. In addition, a neuropeptide, gastrin-releasing peptide (GRP), which also may be released from enteric nerve fibers, acts as a potent stimulus for secretion of gastrin from the G-cells (9). Physiologically, gastrin is released from G-cells in response to the presence of food in the stomach. Food stimulates gastrin secretion both through a reflex response to distention and through a direct action of peptides and amino acids on the G-cell (10). Gastrin is a true hormone, since it is secreted directly into the blood and must be transported by the systemic circulation to its target cells.

A principal target for gastrin is the ECL cell of the fundic mucosa. The ECL cell possesses a peptide receptor, the gastrin or CCK-B subtype peptide receptor, which has a high affinity for gastrin (11,12). Binding of gastrin to this receptor stimulates the ECL cell to release histamine, which in turn activates the parietal cell through the histamine H_2 receptor (13). While it has been suggested that gastrin may stimulate the parietal cell directly, most studies indicate that gastrin stimulated acid secretion primarily, if not exclusively, through release of histamine from the ECL cells. The role of the CCK-B receptor on the parietal cell is not clear, but may be more related to maintaining a differentiated state, or activation of acid secretion by this receptor may require a permissive elevation of cAMP. Some of these ideas are shown in figure 19.

A third pathway for neural stimulation of acid secretion also involves the ECL cells. Acetylcholine, released from enteric nerve fibers in the fundic mucosa, diffuses to the ECL cells where it stimulates the release of histamine. The cholinergic receptor on the ECL cell is different from that on the parietal cell, being more sensitive to M_1 muscarinic antagonists such as pirenzepine (11). An ECL cell is shown closely associated with a parietal cell in the electron micrograph of figure 20.

The central role of histamine in mediating peripheral stimulation of acid secretion was suggested by the ability of histamine H_2 receptor antagonists to inhibit cholinergic and gastrin-stimulated secretion (14). A critical piece of evidence that had been missing was the identification of the source of gastric histamine and how acetylcholine and gastrin elicit the release of this histamine. The recent development of preparations of isolated ECL cells has confirmed that this cell type is the source of gastric histamine and has allowed identification of some of the mechanisms responsible for histamine release (11,12).

ECL cells are one of the several types of endocrine cell found in the oxyntic glands of the stomach. The ECL cell was identified 20 years ago by electron microscopy as a small, 10-μm diameter, cell distributed sparsely along the basal surfaces of the parietal and peptic cells with no connection to the lumen of the gland (15,16). This cell is distinguished from other endocrine cells by virtue of the characteristic granules within its cytoplasm. Many of the granules contain an eccen-

(text continues on p. 52)

FIG. 18. Neural mechanisms for stimulation of acid secretion. The major pathways are illustrated. The central nervous component is mediated via the vagus nerve which synapses with ganglion cells of the enteric nervous system (ENS). The ENS stimulates acid secretion directly by releasing acetylcholine within the fundic mucosa binding to the M_3 receptor of the parietal cell and indirectly by stimulating the enterochromaffin-like (ECL) cell to release histamine. The ENS acts also to stimulate gastrin release from the G-cell of the antrum. Gastrin in turn stimulates release of histamine from the ECL cell. The histamine released from the ECL cell is the major, but not the only, direct stimulant of acid secretion by the parietal cell when it binds to the H_2 receptor.

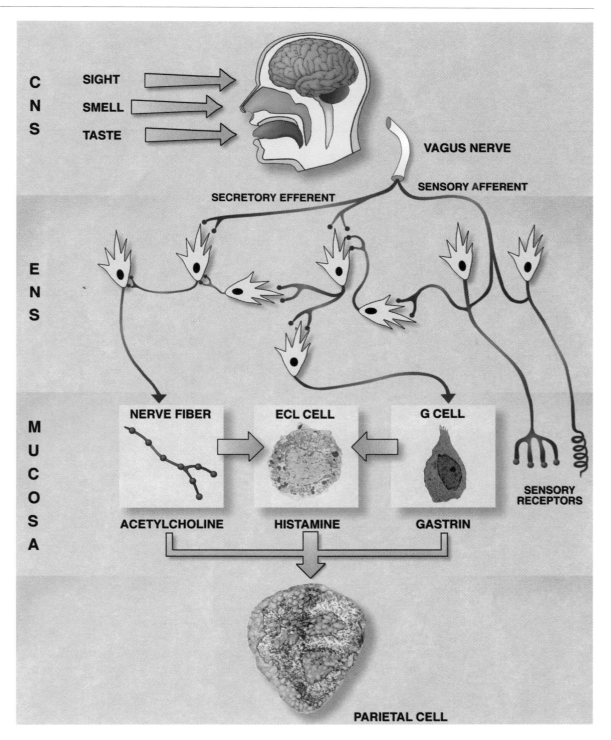

CNS

SIGHT

SMELL

TASTE

VAGUS NERVE

SECRETORY EFFERENT   SENSORY AFFERENT

ENS

MUCOSA

NERVE FIBER	ECL CELL	G CELL

SENSORY
RECEPTORS

ACETYLCHOLINE   HISTAMINE   GASTRIN

PARIETAL CELL

FIG. 18

FIG. 19. An expanded illustration of the peripheral regulation of acid secretion. The presence of food in the stomach (i.e., peptides and amino acids) stimulates the G-cell of the antrum to release gastrin into the circulation. Gastrin travels via the blood to the oxyntic mucosa, where it activates the ECL cell to release histamine. Acetylcholine, released from enteric nerve fibers, stimulates both the ECL cell and the parietal cell. The histamine released from the ECL cell and the acetylcholine released from the nerve fibers stimulate acid secretion by the parietal cell. The release of gastrin is inhibited by the presence of acid (pH <3) in the antrum acting both directly on the G-cell and indirectly through release of somatostatin from the D-cell.

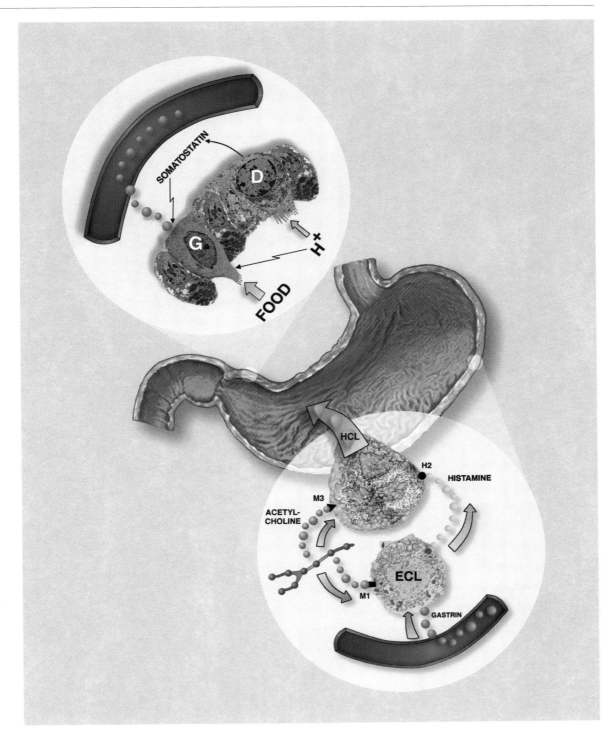

FIG. 19

FIG. 20. A scanning electron micrograph of a gastric gland, highlighting the presence of ECL cells associated with parietal cells.

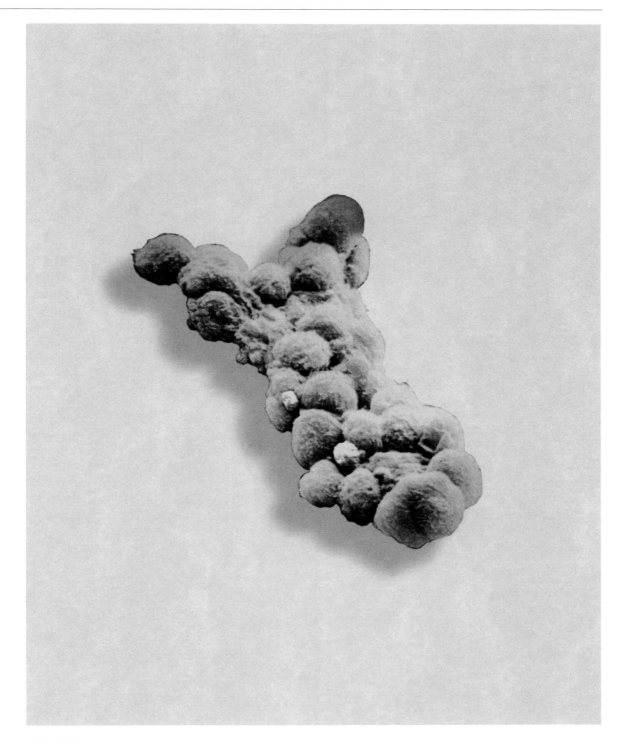

FIG. 20

tric, electron-dense core within a hollow, membrane-bounded vesicle. Using histo-chemical techniques (17,18), these granules have been shown to contain histamine, while the histamine-synthesizing enzyme histidine-decarboxylase has been shown to be located in the cytoplasm of ECL cells. Among the various histamine pools in the gastric mucosa, the pool in the ECL cells has been suggested to be the major source for mediating food- or neural-induced acid secretion (17,19).

Recent studies of isolated ECL cells have provided direct evidence that this cell is responsible for local histamine release when properly stimulated (11). When living ECL cells are stained with the fluorescent pH-sensitive dye acridine orange, the cytoplasmic granules appear bright red, as shown in figure 21, indicating that they are acidic. This acidity is characteristic of the cytoplasmic granules visible in the EM of figure 22, which accumulate bioactive amine compounds, such as chromaffin cells of the adrenal gland (20). Identification of the ECL cell as the source of gastric histamine represents one of the final pieces of evidence confirming a central role for histamine in the stimulation of acid secretion.

The ECL cell releases histamine in response to several stimuli. A model for stimulation of the ECL cell is presented in figure 23. The most important of these, in terms of pathways for stimulating acid secretion, are acetylcholine and gastrin (11), as described above. Histamine which is released from the ECL cell diffuses to nearby parietal cells, where it binds to a histamine H_2 receptor, leading to activation of the parietal cell. The amount of histamine released by the ECL cell is very small. This is sufficient to fully activate nearby parietal cells but too little to cause a systemic response or even a response in cells beyond about 100 µm distant from the ECL cell. The estimated amount of histamine that is released from a single ECL cell (11) is on the order of 1–10 fmol (10^{-15} mol). Because it exerts its effect only at a local level, the histamine released by the ECL cell is termed a paracrine agent. The inability to detect histamine in the venous outflow from the stomach was a major argument against histamine's being an important endogenous stimulus. The description of paracrine or local actions of regulatory substances has now eliminated this argument. There are also feedback pathways inhibiting histamine release from the ECL cell, such as somatostatin acting via a type 2 somatostatin receptor and histamine itself acting via an H_3 receptor.

(text continues on p. 58)

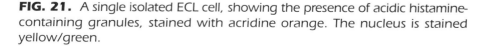

FIG. 21. *A single isolated ECL cell, showing the presence of acidic histamine-containing granules, stained with acridine orange. The nucleus is stained yellow/green.*

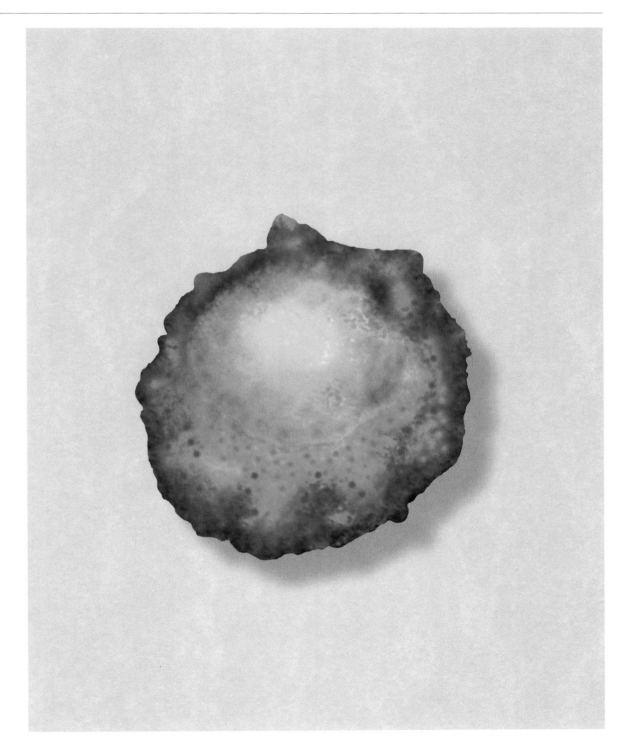

FIG. 21

FIG. 22. A transmission electron micrograph of an isolated ECL cell, showing the acidic vacuoles, colored red, that contain the histamine used for stimulation of acid secretion by the parietal cell.

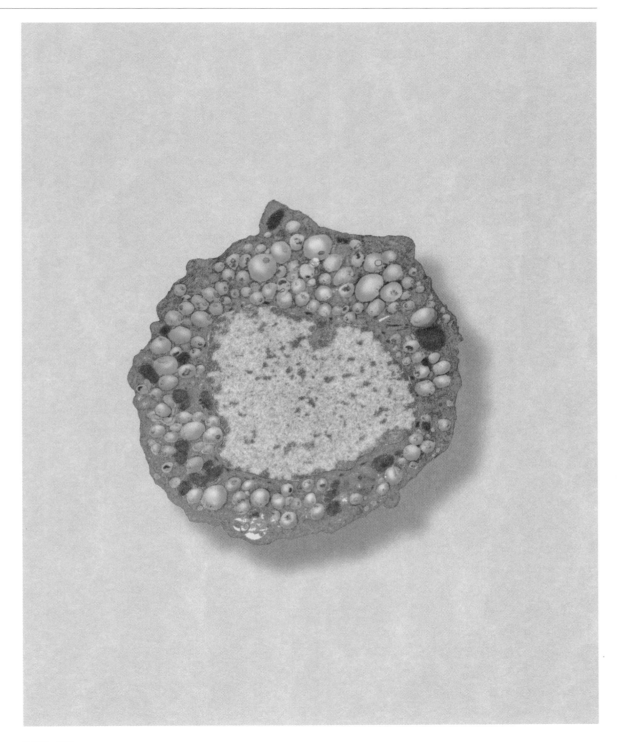

FIG. 22

FIG. 23. The receptors stimulating ECL secretion of histamine, the gastrin receptor, which is a CCK B subtype, and the acetylcholine receptor, perhaps a muscarinic 1 subtype. Both receptors activate histamine release by elevation of intracellular calcium. Not illustrated is the epinephrine receptor, which is a ß-adrenergic subtype working via elevation of cAMP inside the cell. This receptor also stimulates histamine release.

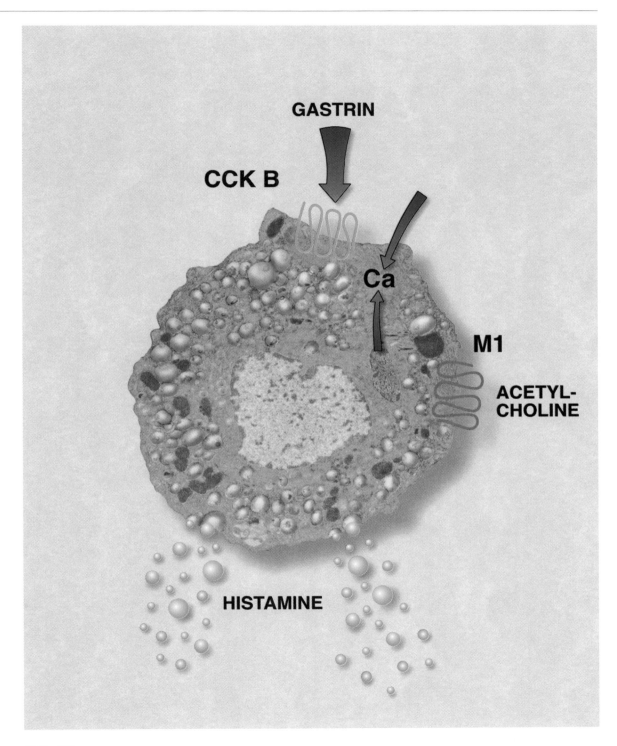

FIG. 23

■ Cellular Stimulation

The primary stimuli acting directly on the parietal cell to stimulate acid secretion are acetylcholine and histamine, as illustrated in figure 24. Of these two, histamine is quantitatively the more important. The action of gastrin on the parietal cell may not be involved directly in acid secretion or may always require the additional presence of a second stimulus of acid secretion.

Histamine acts at a specific subtype of histamine receptor present on the parietal cell, the H_2 receptor (13,14). This receptor subtype differs from the H_1 and H_3 histamine receptors. This receptor is blocked by specific H_2 antagonists but not by the more common anti-H_1 antagonists or by compounds that inhibit the H_3 receptor.

The H_2 receptor protein is a member of a large family of receptors which are associated with guanine nucleotide-binding proteins, or G proteins (21). The G protein acts to couple the receptor protein to enzymes or ion channels which activate the intracellular second messengers leading to cell function. In the case of the histamine H_2 receptor, the G protein activates the enzyme adenylate cyclase, which converts ATP to cyclic AMP (22). The increase of cellular cyclic AMP then leads to activation of the acid pumps by stimulation of phosphorylation of intracellular proteins.

Acetylcholine acts directly on the parietal cell through binding to a M_3 subtype of muscarinic receptor (7,8). The M_3 receptor also is a member of the G protein–associated receptor family. Activation of the M_3 receptor on the parietal cell leads to an increase of intracellular calcium, $[Ca^{+}]i$. The increase of $[Ca^{+}]i$ is biphasic (7). There is an initial rapid, but transient, increase due to release of calcium from intracellular storage sites, located in the endoplasmic reticulum. Simultaneously there is a slower, but sustained, rise due to entry of calcium from the extracellular space through receptor-activated channels. The second phase is required for activation of the acid pumps of the parietal cell, the first phase for Ca-dependent stimulation of Ca entry.

FIG. 24. A model of stimulation of the parietal cell. The H_2 receptor when activated by histamine stimulates adenylate cyclase by activation of G proteins, forming cAMP. The muscarinic M_3 receptor on the surface of the parietal cell is stimulated by acetylcholine, activating other G proteins which activate calcium release from intracellular stores by formation of inositol trisphosphate, and calcium entry from interstitial fluid through a calcium entry pathway. Calcium and cAMP activate a set of protein phosphokinases which drive movement of the pump into the secretory canaliculus and activate a K^+, Cl^- pathway in the canalicular membrane.

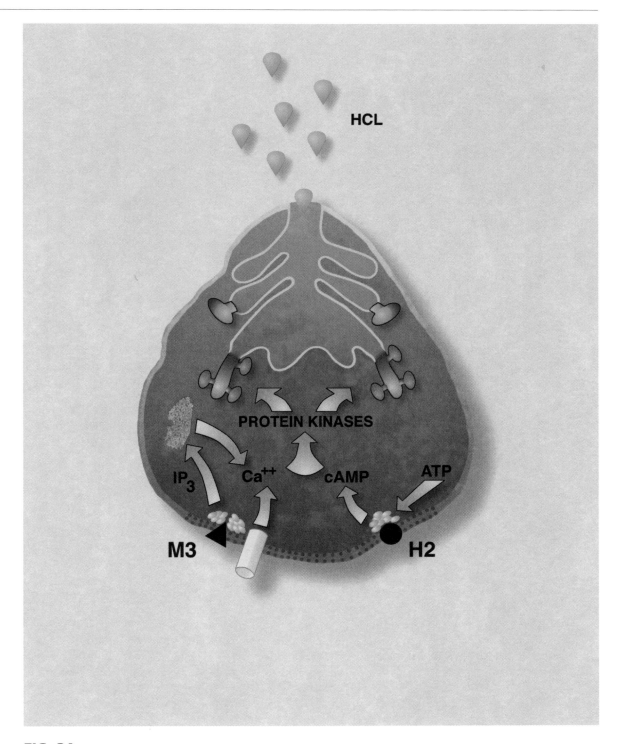

FIG. 24

The two intracellular second messengers cyclic AMP and calcium are capable of activating the acid pumps independently. However, under most conditions it is thought that histamine and acetylcholine interact to produce a greater stimulation than either one alone. This synergism or potentiation most likely occurs by interaction of the intracellular targets of cyclic AMP and calcium.

The molecular mechanisms by which the second messengers activate the acid pumps are not known in detail. It is reasonably certain that the second messengers initially activate one or more protein kinases, enzymes which phosphorylate proteins. Possible protein kinases include one which is cyclic AMP–dependent, protein kinase A, and two which are activated by calcium, protein kinase C and calcium-calmodulin kinase. Based on the known events associated with activation of the acid pumps (Section I), the action of the protein kinases must lead to recruitment of pumps into the secretory canaliculus and to an increase in the permeability of the secretory membrane to KCl. It is known that the acid pump itself is not a substrate for the protein kinases.

Cellular Inhibition of Acid Secretion

The major inhibitory influence on parietal cell function is somatostatin, released mostly from the fundic D-cell. This hormone interacts with a somatostatin type 2 receptor on the ECL cell to ablate histamine release stimulated by gastrin or other agonists (32). Other inhibitors have been suggested such as EGF or TGFα but their physiological role is less well defined. Inhibition via somatostatin therefore depends on somatostatin release from the D-cell, stimulated for example by CGRP, calcitonin gene–related peptide, released from nerve terminals, or by feedback stimulation by gastrin (33).

Control of Acidity

Stimulation of the parietal cells alone is not an efficient regulatory system for control of acidity within the stomach lumen. In addition to stimulation there must be mechanisms to detect acidity and to modulate the level of stimulation or directly alter the secretion of acid in order to avoid excess secretion. The major known mechanism for control of gastric acidity is through feedback regulation of gastrin release by intragastric pH (23). This mechanism is illustrated in figure 19.

Reduction of the intragastric pH below 3 inhibits the release of gastrin from the G-cells of the antrum (2). The exact mechanism of this inhibition is not fully understood but likely involves two possible pathways. The G-cells of the antrum are classified as 'open' type cells in that the apical surfaces are in direct contact with the gastric lumen (24). As such, the apical surface could serve to detect pH directly and alter gastrin release appropriately. A second possible mechanism for pH regulation of gastrin release is indirect through the antral D-cells. D-cells synthesize and release somatostatin, which is known to be a potent inhibitor of gastrin release by the G-cell (25). Since the D-cells of the antrum also are of the 'open' type, it is possible that these cells sense pH and release somatostatin in response to increasing acidity. The D-cells possess long cytoplasmic processes which extend to several nearby cells (26), including G-cells, suggesting that somatostatin is released locally as a paracrine agent rather than circulating in the blood as a true hormone. One or both of these mechanisms then accounts for the inhibition of gastrin release at low intragastric pH. The actual pH at the sensor system regulating inhibition of gastrin release is not known, since luminal pH, unless high buffer concentrations are used, does not necessarily correspond to surface pH.

Reduction of circulating gastrin levels at low intragastric pH leads to reduced histamine release by the ECL cells of the fundus and thus to reduced acid secretion. Although gastrin stimulation of the ECL cell is only one of the pathways for stimulating the parietal cell, it appears to be the most important factor for control of acid secretion by the peripheral pathway. This is consistent with the observation that cholinergic stimulation of histamine release from the ECL cell is less effective than gastrin stimulation (11, 27). Hence reduction of plasma gastrin will decrease parietal cell stimulation.

The feedback control of gastrin release by intragastric pH has physiological implications for anti-secretory therapy. The use of anti-secretory strategies such as highly selective vagotomy, fundectomy, or administration of H_2 receptor antagonists or pump inhibitors (as discussed in Section III) results in elevation of intragastric pH to levels above 3 but does not remove the peripheral stimuli for gastrin release. This interferes with the feedback regulation of gastrin secretion and often leads to hypergastrinemia (28,29). The elevation of plasma gastrin observed in man is small even during long-term anti-secretory treatment (29,30). The hypergastrinemia observed in man under these conditions is considered to be of little or no clinical significance (27).

REFERENCES

1. Tache, Y.: Central nervous system regulation of acid secretion. In, Johnson, L. R. (ed): Physiology of the Gastrointestinal Tract. 2nd ed., Vol. 2, Raven Press, New York, USA, p. 911, 1987.

2. Hirschowitz, B.: Neural and hormonal control of gastric secretion. In, Handbook of Physiology, Section 6, The Gastrointestinal Tract. Vol. 3, Oxford University Press, New York, p. 127, 1989.

3. Debas, H. T. and Lloyd K.C.K.: Peripheral regulation of gastric acid secretion. In, Johnson, L. R. (ed): Physiology of the Gastrointestinal Tract. 3rd ed., Vol 2, Raven Press, New York, USA, p. 1185, 1994.

4. Hoffman, H. H., and Schnitzlein, N. N.: The number of vagus fibers in man. Anat. Rec. 139, 429, 1969.

5. Wood, J. D.: Physiology of the enteric nervous system. In, Johnson, L. R. (ed.): Physiology of the Gastrointestinal Tract. 3rd ed., Vol. 1, Raven Press, New York, USA, p. 423, 1994.

6. Costa, M., Furness, J. B., and Llewellyn-Smith, I. J.: Histochemistry of the enteric nervous system. In, Johnson, L. R. (ed.): Physiology of the Gastrointestinal Tract. 2nd ed., Vol. 1, Raven Press, New York, USA, p. 1, 1987.

7. Wilkes, J. M., Kajimura, M., Scott, D. R., Hersey, S. J., and Sachs, G.: Muscarinic responses of gastric parietal cells. J. Membrane Biol. 122, 97, 1991.

8. Kajimura, M., Reuben, M., and Sachs, G.: The muscarinic receptor gene expressed in rabbit parietal cells is the M_3 subtype. Gastroenterology 103, 870, 1992.

9. Schepp, W., Prinz, C., Hakanson, R., Schusdziarra, V., and Classen, M.: Effects of bombesin-like peptides on isolated rat gastric G-cells. Reg. Peptides 28, 241, 1990.

10. Lichtenberger, L. M.: Importance of food in the regulation of gastrin release and formation. Am. J. Physiol. 243, G429, 1982.

11. Prinz, C., Kajimura, M., Scott, D. R., Mercier, F., Helander, H. F., and Sachs, G.: Histamine secretion from rat enterochromaffin-like cells. Gastroenterology 105, 449, 1993.

12. Kopin, A. S., Y. M. Lee, E. W. McBride, L. J. Miller, M. Lu, H. Y. Lin, L. F. Kolakowski,Jr., and M. Beinborn.: (1992) Expression cloning and characterization of the canine parietal cell gastrin receptor. Proc. Natl. Acad. Sci. U. S. A. 89, 3605-3609, 1992.

13. Gantz, I., Schaeffer, M., DelValle, J., Logsdon, C., Campbell, V., Uhler, M., and Yamada, T.: Molecular cloning of a gene encoding the histamine H_2-receptor. Proc. Natl. Acad. Sci. USA, 488, 429, 1991.

14. Black, J. W., Duncan, W. A. M., Durant, C. J., Ganellin, C. R., and Parsons, M. E.: Definition and antagonism of histamine H_2 receptors. Nature 236, 385, 1972.

15. Hakanson, R., Owman, C. H., Sporong, B., and Sundler, F.: Electron microscopic identification of the histamine-storing argyrophil (enterochromaffin-like) cells in the rat stomach. Z. Zellforschung Mikroskop. Anatomie 122, 460, 1971.

16. Capella, C., Vassallo, G., and Solcia, E.: Light and electron microscopic identification of the histamine-storing agyrophil (ECL) cell in murine stomach and of its equivalent in other mammals. Zeitschrift Zellforschung 118, 68, 1971.

17. Hakanson, R., Boettcher, G., Ekblad, F., Panula, P., Simonsson, M., Dohlsten, M., Hallberg, T., and Sundler, F.: Histamine in endocrine cells in the stomach. Histochemistry 86, 5, 1986.

18. Simonsson, M., Eriksson, S., Hakanson, R., Lind, T., Loenroth, L., Lundell, L., O'Connor, D. T., and Sundler, F.: Endocrine cells in the human oxyntic mucosa. Scand. J. Gastroenterol. 23, 1089, 1988.

19. Rangachari, P .K.: Histamine, mercurial messenger in the gut. Am. J. Physiol. 262, G1, 1992.

20. Johnson, R. G., Carty, S. E., and Scarpa, A.: Coupling of H^+ gradients to cathecholamine transport in chromaffin granules. Ann. NY Acad. Sci. 456, 254, 1985.

21. Dohlman, H. G., Thorner, J., Caron, M. G., and Lefkowitz, R. J..: G-proteins. Ann. Rev. Biochem. 60, 653, 1991.

22. Chew, C. S., Hersey, S. J., Sachs, G., and Berglindh, T.: Histamine responsiveness of isolated gastric glands. Am. J. Physiol. 238, G312, 1980.

23. Walsh, J. H.: Gastrointestinal hormones, in Physiology of the Gastrointestinal Tract, edited by L.R. Johnson, Raven Press, p 1 , 1994

24. Fujita, T., and Kobayashi, S.: Structure and function of gut endocrine cells. Int. Rev. Cytol. 6, 187, 1977.

25. Seal, A. M., Yamada, T. and Debas, H. T.: Somatostatin 14 and 28, clearance and potency on gastric function in dogs. Am. J. Physiol. 143, G97, 1982.

26. Larsson, H., Golterman, N., DeMagistris, L., Rehfeld, J. F., and Schwartz, T. W.: Somatostatin cell processes as pathways for paracrine secretion. Science 205, 1393, 1979.

27. Gerber, J. G., and Payne, N. A.: The role of gastric secretagogues in regulating gastric histamine release in vivo. Gastroenterology 102, 403, 1992.

28. Lind, T., Cederberg, C., Olausson, M., and Olbe, L.: 24-hour intragastric acidity and plasma gastrin after omeprazole treatment and after proximal gastric vagotomy in duodenal ulcer patients. Gastroenterology 99, 1593, 1990.

29. Brunner, G. H. G., Lamberts, R., and Creutzfeld, W.: Efficacy and safety of omeprazole in the long-term treatment of peptic ulcer and reflux oesophagitis resistant to ranitidine. Digestion 47(Suppl 1):64, 1990.

30. Kohn, A., Annibale, B., Prantera, C., et al.: Reversible sustained increase of gastrin and gastric acid secretion in a subgroup of duodenal ulcer patients on long term treatment with H_2 antagonists. J. Clin. Gastroenterol. 134, 284, 1991.

31. Freston, J. W.: Clinical significance of hypergastrinemia. Digestion 51, 102, 1992.

32. Prinz C, Sachs G, Walsh J, Coy D, and Wu V.: The somatostatin receptor subtype on rat enterochromaffin-like cells. Gastroenterology, 107, 1067, 1994.

33. Lewin M.J.M.: The somatostatin receptor in the GI tract. Annu. Rev. Physiol. 54, 455,1992.

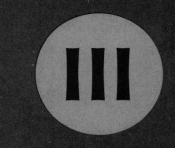
Actions of
Anti-Secretory
Agents

OVERVIEW

Reduction of gastric acidity is a primary goal in the management of acid-related disorders whether associated with *Helicobacter* infection or not. Currently available options include antacids, receptor antagonists, and acid pump inhibitors.

Antacids produce prompt but brief symptom relief by neutralizing acid already present in the stomach. Therapy with antacids requires frequent administration of large doses and is not practical for healing or maintenance therapy in frank ulcer disease. Antacids do not reduce the acidity of the gastric wall, since they do not penetrate the lumen of the gastric gland.

Receptor antagonists inhibit acid formation by blocking specific steps in the pathways which regulate secretion by the parietal cells. Such antagonists include those selective for muscarinic acetylcholine receptors and those selective for histamine H_2 receptors. Of such receptor antagonists, only the H_2 receptor antagonists have found widespread clinical application due to their efficacy and relative freedom from side effects. Due to their short plasma half life, the currently available receptor antagonists have a short duration of action, and their ability to inhibit acid secretion may be compromised by increased levels of agonists or the presence of alternative pathways for stimulation.

Acid pump inhibitors act directly on the H^+,K^+-ATPase, the final step in acid secretion. These agents are highly selective and inhibit secretion regardless of the level or nature of the stimuli acting on the parietal cells. The acid pump inhibitor omeprazole belongs to a class of chemicals called the substituted benzimidazoles.

Omeprazole is a prodrug. Omeprazole accumulates selectively in the acidic spaces generated within the secretory canaliculus of the parietal cell, becomes activated, and forms a covalent complex with the H^+,K^+-ATPase resulting in inhibition of the active acid pump. As additional acid pumps become active, repeated doses of omeprazole inhibit more of the H^+,K^+-ATPase molecules. New pump molecules also are being synthesized, and a steady-state level of inhibition is achieved in humans within three to five days on once-a-day dosing. More frequent administration leads to greater steady-state suppression of acid secretion. Even though it requires some time to reach a steady-state level of inhibition, the efficacy of the pump inhibitors is such that superior symptom relief is achieved as compared to H_2 antagonists. The unique chemistry of substituted benzimidazoles accounts for their high selectivity and relatively long duration of action.

This section is illustrated in figures 25 through 32.

ANTI-SECRETORY AGENTS

Reduction in gastric acidity is a desirable therapeutic goal. The extent and duration of gastric pH elevation which is optimum for symptom relief and healing varies with the specific disorder, as discussed in Section IV. However, any effective strategy requires rapid symptom relief and healing, broad spectrum of efficacy, freedom from untoward side effects, and stability of acidity control. Prior to the 1970's the medical options available were dietary and postural measures, non-selective anti-cholinergics, and antacids. Of these, only the antacids persist generally as a therapeutic approach, and these are reserved for the mildest forms of acid-related disorders and for relief of symptoms, not for healing. Over the past two decades, treatment of acid-related disease has been revolutionized by the development of two classes of drugs, H_2 receptor antagonists and acid pump inhibitors. Both classes are targeted to the parietal cell and act to reduce acid secretion by this cell, in contrast to the antacids, which do not affect parietal cell acid secretion directly. However, the receptor antagonists and the pump inhibitors are quite distinct in their mechanism of action, and this difference has important implications for their therapeutic properties. The known sites of action for the principal classes of antisecretory agents are illustrated in figure 25. The physician has several choices available for inhibition of acid secretion.

FIG. 25. The sites of action of various agents designed to reduce intragastric acidity. Antacids are shown neutralizing secreted acid. The selective muscarinic antagonist pirenzepine perhaps inhibits histamine release from the ECL cell that is stimulated by acetylcholine. The non-selective muscarinic antagonist atropine blocks both acetylcholine stimulation of histamine release and its direct stimulation of the parietal cell. The H_2 antagonists compete with histamine at the H_2 receptor on the parietal cell. Omeprazole inhibits the active gastric acid pump.

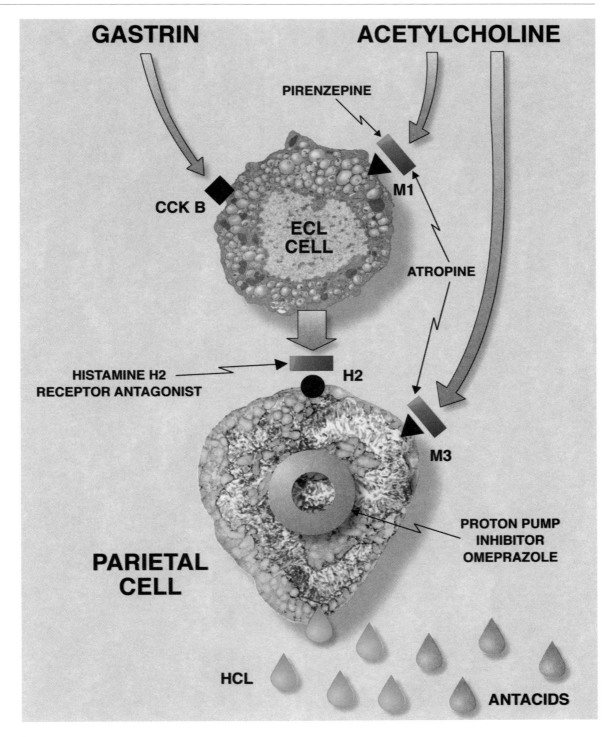

GASTRIN

ACETYLCHOLINE

PIRENZEPINE

CCK B

ECL CELL

M1

ATROPINE

HISTAMINE H2 RECEPTOR ANTAGONIST

H2

M3

PROTON PUMP INHIBITOR OMEPRAZOLE

PARIETAL CELL

HCL

ANTACIDS

FIG. 25

■ Antacids

Antacids have been used for centuries for the symptomatic relief of ulcer disease and esophagitis. These agents do not alter the acid secretory mechanism itself but only neutralize acid already present in the stomach. Although antacids are used as a conservative approach to reducing gastric acidity which provides symptom relief, they have several disadvantages. Their duration of action is very brief, requiring frequent, 6-8 times daily, administration of high doses. Because of this, antacids are poorly suited to long-term usage and are prone to complications resulting from inadequate control of secretion. There are also complications due to the antacids themselves. Complications include diarrhea, particularly with magnesium salts, disorders of mineral balance, and alkalosis (1). The last symptom is due mainly to the fact that neutralized acid becomes unavailable for reabsorption or reaction with pancreatic bicarbonate, which is necessary for maintaining normal acid-base balance.

Under normal circumstances gastric acidity suppresses gastrin release from the antrum of the stomach (see Section II). Antacids interfere with this regulatory mechanism and may result in 'rebound' hyperacidity when the antacid is no longer present in the stomach. Additionally, the high calcium content of specific antacids can directly stimulate the antral G-cell to release excess gastrin.

The pharmacological properties of antacids, therefore, suggest that they are not suitable as the sole therapy for reliable management of acid secretion in acid-related disease. Their clinical use should be reserved for symptom relief or as adjunctive therapy at the beginning of medical treatment. If a patient continues to use antacids during medical therapy, his or her acid secretion is not being controlled adequately by the therapy chosen.

■ Anticholinergics

The earliest attempts to inhibit acid secretion by blocking receptors involved the use of atropine to inhibit stimulation by the vagus nerve. Atropine is a non-selective antagonist of muscarinic cholinergic receptors. Because muscarinic receptors are distributed throughout the body, atropine produces a variety of side effects such as blurred vision and dry mouth (2).

Recognition that muscarinic receptors occur in distinct subtypes, at least five of which have been identified, has prompted the development of subtype-selective antagonists for various diseases. At present there are no marketed antagonists selective for the M_3 subtype receptor, which is present on the parietal cell. However, the M_1 subtype antagonist pirenzepine has shown promise in inhibiting acid secretion with fewer of the side effects found with the non-selective antagonist atropine (3). The efficacy of M_1 receptor antagonists is likely related to the role of this receptor subtype in mediating signal transmission in the ENS and perhaps in stimulating the ECL cells to release histamine. Since histamine release from the ECL cells is stimulated also by non-cholinergic mechanisms, e.g., gastrin, the M_1 receptor antagonists are found to inhibit only 50–60% of meal-stimulated acid secretion (2). This probably is not sufficient to raise intragastric pH to a therapeutically effective level in many patients.

■ Histamine H$_2$ Receptor Antagonists

The synthesis and development of selective antagonists for the histamine 2 receptor by James Black and his colleagues (4) is a landmark in the medical management of acid-related disorders. Cimetidine (Tagamet®), the first clinically effective H$_2$ receptor antagonist, has been joined by a family of similar drugs, including ranitidine (Zantac®), famotidine (Pepcid®), and nizatidine (Axid®). An important element in the development of these agents was the observation that the selectivity for the H$_2$ receptor depends upon the nature of the alkyl side chain rather than the imidazole ring of histamine. In contrast, the structural requirements for the H$_1$ receptor antagonists depended on modification of the imidazole ring rather than the side chain(5). Both H$_1$ and H$_2$ receptor antagonists are competitive, hence are displaced by histamine from their binding site.

The currently available H$_2$ receptor antagonists differ in their potency, but not in their fundamental mechanism of action resulting in similar efficacy. These drugs competitively inhibit the binding of histamine at the H$_2$ subtype receptor. Although H$_2$ subtype histamine receptors are found in the heart, kidneys, and lymphocytes, the major pharmacological effect of the H$_2$ receptor antagonists is due to blockade of the histamine receptor of the gastric parietal cell. Few side effects have been found that can be related to H$_2$ antagonist blockade of H$_2$ receptors elsewhere in the body.

Thus, although H$_2$ receptor antagonists are effective in blocking histamine-driven acid secretion, they are only partially effective in blocking the acid secretion dependent on cholinergic stimulation, which must be an important element in stimulation of daytime acid secretion (6,7). This spectrum of action is consistent with the known mechanisms responsible for activating the parietal cell, as described in Section II. The stimulation of acid secretion by food in the stomach is mediated by release of gastrin from the antral G-cells, and the action of gastrin, in turn, is mediated by the release of histamine from the ECL cells of the oxyntic glands. In contrast, vagal stimulation due to sensory input activates the parietal cell by a direct action of acetylcholine released from nerve fibers acting at an M$_3$ muscarinic receptor. In addition there is stimulation of release of histamine from the ECL cell. An H$_2$ receptor antagonist will therefore block gastrin-stimulated acid secretion and that component of acid secretion due to vagal stimulation of histamine release from the ECL cell. The antagonist will not, however, affect the direct stimulation of the M$_3$ receptor on the parietal cell. Hence vagally mediated acid secretion will be relatively insensitive to H$_2$ receptor antagonists.

The efficacy and duration of action of the H$_2$ receptor antagonists relates to their mechanism of action as competitive antagonists at the H$_2$ receptor. These drugs are effective only as long as their plasma concentration exceeds that which is required to compete with the endogenous histamine at the receptor. Since the plasma half life of the current H$_2$ receptor antagonists is on the order of 2–4 hours (8), their duration of action is relatively short. This property requires taking multiple daily doses (bid for Du, qid for erosive esophagitis) to obtain the stable reduction in gastric acidity over a 24-hr period that seems optimal for healing of many acid-dependent lesions.

The efficacy of H$_2$ receptor antagonists depends also on the intensity of endogenous stimulation. Changes in the level of alternative pathways for stimulation will alter the effectiveness of these competitive inhibitors and may lead to acid secretory breakthrough or tachyphylaxis (9). There is in addition the liability of acid rebound, wherein the rate of acid secretion increases following withdrawal of medication. This is particularly likely when high-frequency, high-dose receptor antagonists are administered, for example for the treatment of GERD.

An additional consideration in the use of H_2 receptor antagonists is the onset of action. Since receptor antagonists act at the initial step in cell activation, full inhibition of acid secretion will not occur immediately when the drug reaches its target. Rather, inhibition is delayed until the existing intracellular activation returns to a resting level and the acid pump is withdrawn from the canalicular membrane. In the case of acid secretion by the parietal cell this would require that the active acid pumps in the secretory canaliculus recycle to their inactive state in the cytoplasmic tubules, a process which requires 30–60 minutes for completion. The rate of inhibition of acid secretion will then depend on the existing activity state of the parietal cell in the gastric mucosa (10).

Another consideration in the use of H_2 antagonist therapy is acid rebound. This occurs in man upon withdrawal of H_2 receptor antagonist therapy (37). Recent data suggest that this may be due, at least in part, to an increased level of the gastric H^+,K^+-ATPase resulting from inhibition of the H_2 receptor (36). This is most likely due to a decreased rate of turnover of the H^+,K^+-ATPase. With constant synthesis, the steady-state level of the pump will increase. This then results in an increased secretory capacity of the gastric mucosa.

As with many receptor active agents, tolerance to H_2 antagonists also occurs. The effectiveness of inhibition with H_2 antagonists declines quite significantly (by as much as 1 pH unit or more) when the first day's effect is compared to the effect on the seventh or the fifteenth day (9). Whether acid rebound or tolerance during treatment with H_2 receptor antagonists is a partial explanation for H_2 resistance in patients is not clear. It seems that increasing the dose or frequency of the H_2 receptor antagonist does not avoid the tolerance and may exacerbate acid rebound, as found in animal experiments (36).

H_2 receptor antagonists have been used clinically for over 20 years with few reported side effects. Some of these drugs are metabolized by the cytochrome P-450 oxidase system in the liver and may interfere with metabolism of other drugs. This may require some adjustment of dosage of the other drugs during H_2 receptor therapy. A few cases of bradycardia have been reported and likely are due to the presence of H_2 receptors in the atria. These few side effects are generally well tolerated and do not pose a serious problem in the clinical use of these agents (8,11).

ACID PUMP INHIBITORS

In the late 1970's, as the H_2 receptor antagonists were changing the clinical management of acid-related disorders, two crucial observations led to the development of a new class of anti-secretory agents, the acid pump inhibitors. First, the gastric H^+,K^+-ATPase was discovered and proposed to be the molecular basis for acid secretion (12,13). Second, a class of chemicals known as substituted benzimidazoles was found to inhibit acid secretion independently of the pathway of stimulation (14). Shortly thereafter it was demonstrated that the substituted benzimidazoles inhibit acid secretion by inhibiting the H^+,K^+-ATPase (14). It was also noted that the compounds were active only when the pump was making acid, resulting in the deduction that these compounds were acid-activated prodrugs (15). Subsequent studies confirmed that the substituted benzimidazoles are highly selective inhibitors of the secreting gastric H^+,K^+-ATPase, and the first acid pump inhibitor, omeprazole (Prilosec®, Losec®, or Antra®), was developed for clinical use in the 1980's.

The success of omeprazole has prompted the synthesis and development of other acid pump inhibitors with a similar mechanism, such as lansoprazole and pantoprazole. While identical in the molecular target, the gastric acid pump, the compounds differ in, for example, acid stability or in the cysteines that react on the α subunit of the pump. The alteration in structure also results in alteration in metabolism, although all three drugs are initially oxidized by the cytochrome P-450 system. It is likely that the differences found in preclinical studies relate rather to the metabolic pathways or acid stability than to their intrinsic activity.

This class of anti-secretory agents has several differences as compared to the H_2 receptor antagonists in terms of control of acid secretion. These distinctions stem directly from the differences in the biological targeting and the chemical mechanism of action of these two classes of anti-secretory agents. The differences result in advantages for acid pump inhibitors in (a) rapid onset of inhibition of acid secretion, (b) lack of tolerance, (c) lack of acid rebound, and (d) independence of the pathway of stimulation of the stomach. In particular, control of daytime acidity appears important in the control of pain in erosive esophagitis and plays a significant role in the healing of duodenal ulcer disease.

Site of Action of Omeprazole

The structure of omeprazole is shown in figure 26. The mechanism of action of omeprazole is best characterized (16,17) as occurring in four stages, absorption, concentration in the parietal cell, activation in the parietal cell, and covalent binding to the catalytic subunit of the H^+,K^+-ATPase. Each of these stages contributes to its selectivity and efficacy, and they are illustrated in figures 27 and 28.

Omeprazole is a weak base with a pK_a of 4.0. At neutral pH the compound is mostly unprotonated and uncharged and can easily cross biological membranes. This property of omeprazole allows for rapid absorption of oral doses and rapid distribution into intracellular compartments.

The concentration of omeprazole by tissues is highly selective owing to its weak base properties. If a weak base enters an acidic space where the pH of the space is lower than the pK_a of the base, it will become mostly protonated and hence positively charged. The protonated form of omeprazole is much less permeable to biological membranes because of this positive charge and, therefore, the compound will concentrate in the acidic space. Because omeprazole has a pK_a of 4, the only space in the body with a pH low enough to concentrate omeprazole is the secretory canaliculus of the parietal cell. The low pH of the secretory canaliculus (pH = 1.0) during acid

(text continues on p. 80)

FIG. 26. The chemical structure of omeprazole.

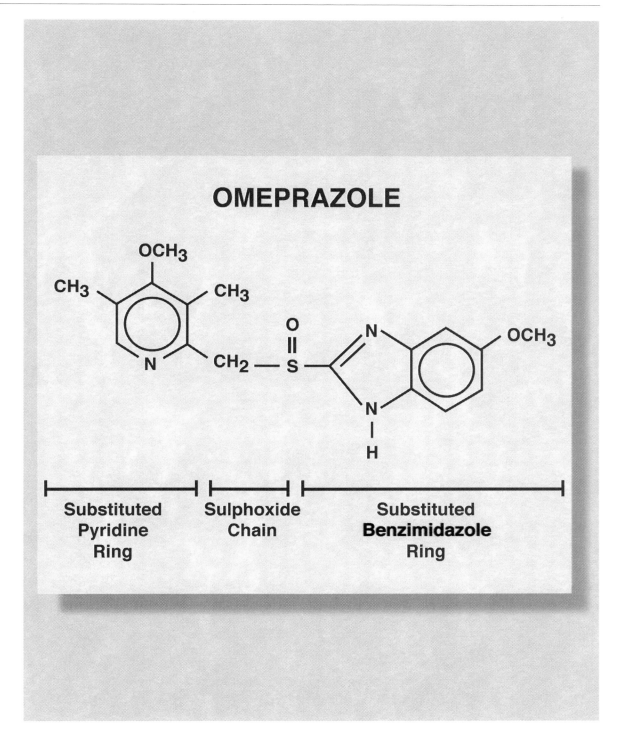

FIG. 26

FIG. 27. The activation of the prodrug, omeprazole. The first step is protonation allowing concentration of the drug exclusively in the active parietal cell's canaliculus. The second step is conversion of the protonated form to the active sulfenamide. The final step is reaction of the sulfenamide with the cysteines available on the active acid pump. C is colored gray, H is white, N is blue, S is yellow, and O is red.

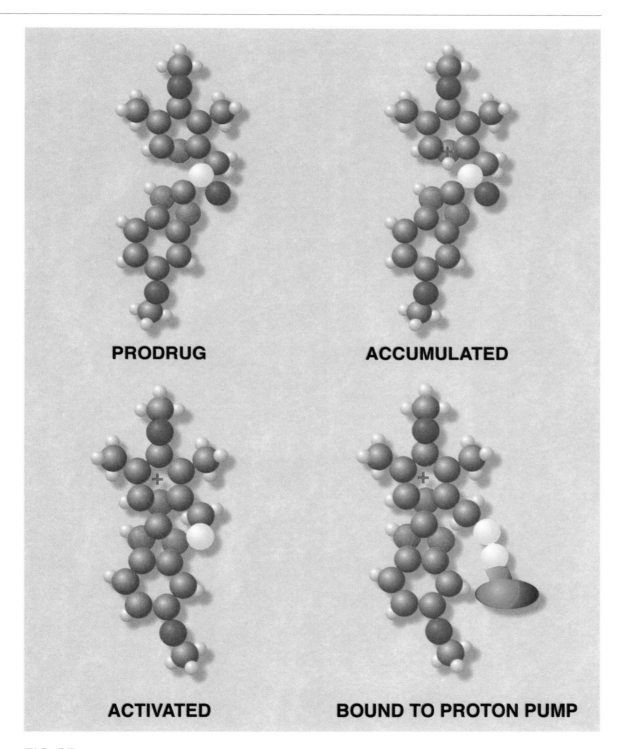

PRODRUG

ACCUMULATED

ACTIVATED

BOUND TO PROTON PUMP

FIG. 27

FIG. 28. An illustration of how omeprazole works in the secreting parietal cell. It enters the cell cytoplasm from the blood, concentrates in the acid space, and then converts to the sulfenamide, the active compound. This reacts with the specific cysteines on the outside surface of the catalytic subunit of the pump.

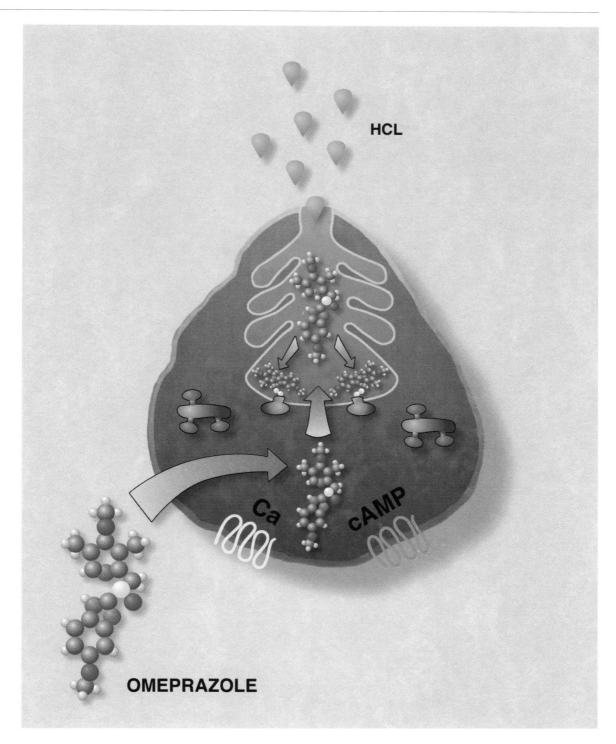

FIG. 28

secretion results in a concentration of omeprazole in the canaliculus about a thousand-fold greater than its level in the blood or other tissues. This selective accumulation of omeprazole by the secretory canaliculus of the parietal cell is the first step critical to the unique target selectivity of omeprazole (15,16).

Omeprazole is a prodrug, that is to say it is not active in the form administered. The prodrug must first be converted in the parietal cell to its active chemical form. The activation of omeprazole involves an acid-catalyzed conversion of the relatively stable methylsulfinyl group to a highly reactive sulfenamide. The conversion to the active form is acid-dependent, occurring rapidly at pH below 3 but slowly at neutral pH, assuring little or no activation in the blood or other tissue spaces. The active sulfenamide is a permanent cation, and the positive charge prevents the activated molecule from leaving the acid space and reacting with intracellular proteins. The conversion to the active cationic form of omeprazole therefore occurs in the acidic space in which the drug is already concentrated, a second element in the specific targeting of the drug. The selective targeting of the drug is shown in the electron micrograph of figure 29.

The chemistry of the proton pump inhibitors (PPI's) is quite subtle. Protonation of the pyridine N drives acid accumulation. However, this N has to deprotonate in order to form the tetracyclic intermediate, the sulfenamide. At the same time the reactivity of the 2C of the benzimidazole has to increase in order to form the active compound. A likely explanation for the mechanism is that there is intramolecular transfer of the pyridine N proton to the benzimidazole N. For this to be achieved, a folded intermediate conformation has to be formed to allow for proton transfer. From the root compound, timoprazole, omeprazole was designed to decrease the pK_a of the pyridine N. A methoxy group was introduced on to the benzimidazole to facilitate cyclization. In the case of pantoprazole, the difluoroethoxy group was intended to produce a more stable form of the prodrug. Whatever the design features, thus far there is little to discriminate between the different approved drugs in terms of clinical results that are not explainable as a function of dose.

An additional factor ensuring the selective targeting of the activated drug is that the half-life of the reactive sulfenamide is pH-dependent, the half-life being

FIG. 29. *An electron microscopic autoradiogram of a stimulated parietal cell treated with radioactive omeprazole, showing that the active pump which binds omeprazole is exclusively in the secretory canaliculus, illustrated by the presence of the precipitated silver grains due to radioactive disintegration over only the canaliculus. The in vivo target of omeprazole is therefore uniquely the acid pump in the secretory canaliculus of the parietal cell.*

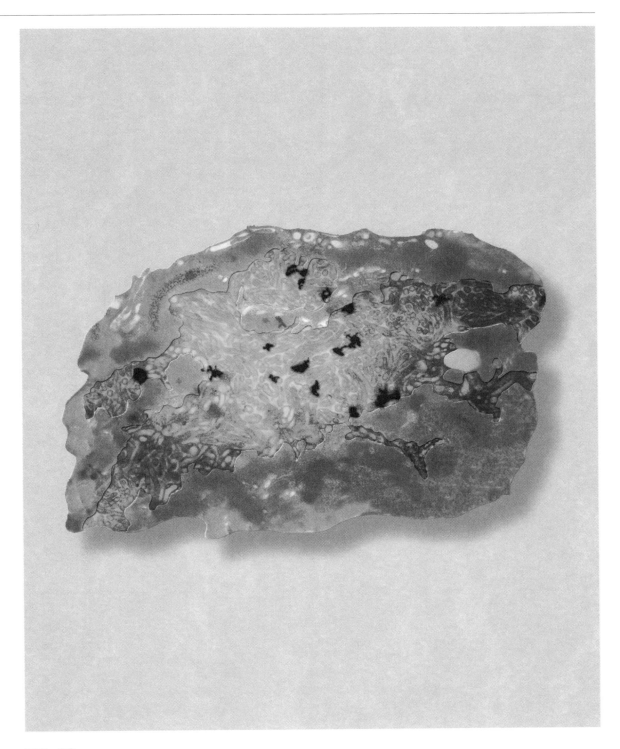

FIG. 29

longer at acidic than at neutral pH. At pH 1 the half life is about 30 minutes, while at pH 7 it is only about 200 milliseconds (16). Thus any activated drug which might escape from the canaliculus is immediately converted to inactive products.

Oral activity of the drug depends absolutely on preventing gastric acid from reacting with the drug before absorption, since it is acid-labile. The current formulation of omeprazole is a micro-encapsulated form, wherein the coating of the individual grains of omeprazole resists acid and omeprazole is not released until a pH of about 6.1 is reached, usually in the upper duodenum.

The sulfenamide is a selective cysteine reagent with respect to biological macromolecules, reacting only with the -SH moiety present on this amino acid. The active form of omeprazole, the sulfenamide, reacts with two cysteine residues in the H^+,K^+-ATPase to form a stable, covalent disulfide derivative (15,18). Formation of the disulfide bond results in covalent inhibition of the transport and enzymatic activity of the acid pump (17).

In principle, the acid-activated form of omeprazole could react with any cysteine that is present in, or accessible from, the acid space in which the active form of the drug is generated. Extensive studies of the sites at which omeprazole is bound have shown that the covalently bound drug is found only in the canaliculus of the gastric parietal cell (see figure 29), confirming the unique targeting of this agent (19). Biochemical analyses further identified the catalytic subunit of the H^+,K^+-ATPase as the only protein which binds the drug (15,18). This is the third element in the specific targeting of omeprazole.

There are 28 cysteines in the catalytic subunit and 9 in the β subunit of the H^+,K^+-ATPase. Of these, 6 cysteines in the β subunit and 3 or 4 cysteines in the α subunit are predicted to be accessible from the extracytoplasmic surface. The cysteines of the β subunit are linked by internal disulfide bonds and therefore not available for stable reaction with the omeprazole sulfenamide. It has been found that omeprazole reacts with only two of the cysteines in the catalytic subunit, as shown in figure 30. One cysteine is located in the extracytosolic loop between transmembrane segments 5 and 6 and a second site is found between transmembrane segments 7 and

FIG. 30. *The critical cysteine site to which omeprazole binds on the catalytic subunit of the ATPase. This is likely to be cysteine number 813 in the linear sequence of the pump, placed in the luminal loop between membrane segments 5 and 6. Given the ion pathway illustrated in figure 16, the formation of the disulfide in this region will block acid transport by the pump. Although cysteine 892 also binds omeprazole, binding to it may not be critical for pump inhibition. Thus the specific target of omeprazole in vivo is cysteine at position 813 of the 1033 amino acids of the α subunit of the H^+,K^+-ATPase, in those pumps that are actively participating in acid secretion by the parietal cell.*

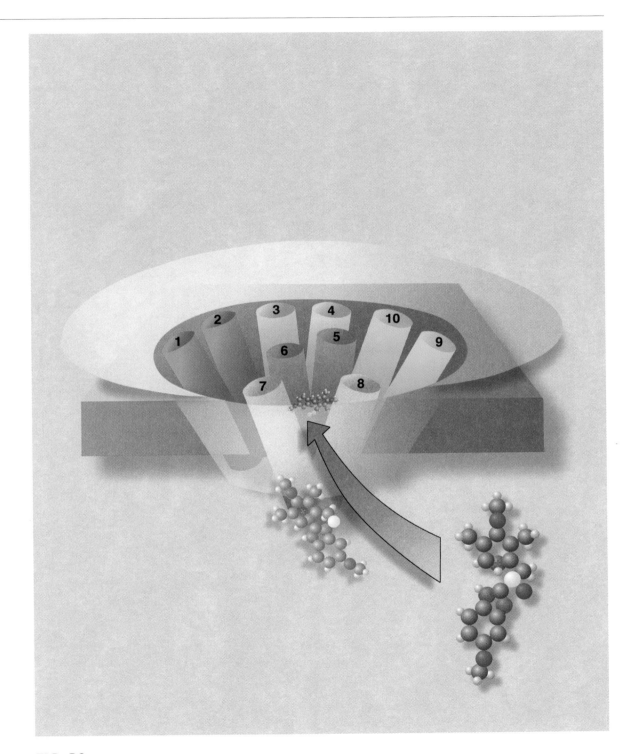

FIG. 30

8 (18). From studies on other substituted benzimidazoles it appears that reaction with only the cysteine between the 5th and 6th membrane segments is sufficient for inhibition of the H^+,K^+-ATPase (21). In effect, the specific target for omeprazole inhibition of acid secretion is a single amino acid, the cysteine at position 813 in the 1033 amino acid chain comprising the acid pump's catalytic subunit (see figure 30). It has been shown that binding of omeprazole to cys 892 is not correlated with inhibition, in contrast to the binding to the cys in TM5/TM6 (40). This is the fourth element in the specific targeting of omeprazole. The other pump inhibitors that have been investigated also target cysteines in the pump, in the case of lansoprazole the cysteines at positions 321, 813, and 892 (20), in the case of pantoprazole, cys 813 and cys 822 (21). These data suggest that it is the common cysteine, cys 813, that is the specific target of the substituted benzimidazole class of pump inhibitor. Recent studies have shown that reaction with cysteine 813 correlates with the rate of omeprazole inhibition of the ATPase, whereas cysteine 892 reacts virtually immediately, and reaction with this cysteine does not correlate well with inhibition (38). Hence it is this single cysteine that is the target of omeprazole.

The unique pharmacological mechanism of omeprazole leads to unique pharmacodyamics (22,23). Similar considerations apply to other proton pump inhibitors. The plasma half life of omeprazole is about 60 minutes in humans. However, since the drug reacts covalently with the pump, the total delivery of the drug to the active pumps is more important than concentration of the drug at a specific point in time. Its effect is therefore more related to the area under the plasma concentration curve than to the peak concentration. Its covalent mechanism provides a duration of action much longer than the plasma half life, in contrast to the reversible antagonists. Therefore a once-a-day regimen will rapidly give secretory suppression over a large part of the day.

The onset of symptom relief depends on the rate and completeness of inhibition of acid secretion. Pump inhibitors inhibit the active pump. Receptor antagonists result in removal of the pump from the canalicular membrane and provide incomplete inhibition of acid secretion except at night. Inhibition of acid secretion by pump inhibition would be expected to be more consistent and therefore provides faster and better symptom relief with the first dose and the results improve with the next dose or two.

Another feature of the action of omeprazole is that, while secretory inhibition is rapid, the anti-secretory action is cumulative, reaching steady state within 48 hrs on once-a-day dosage in humans (23). With the first dose, a fraction of the pumps in the stomach is inactive and hence will not be inhibited. The fraction that is active is covalently blocked. With the second dose, additional pumps are activated and these will now be blocked by omeprazole. At the same time new pumps are being synthesized in the parietal cell, and perhaps there is also some loss of drug from the pump. The fraction of these pumps that are active will be inhibited by the second dose also. The final steady state of acid inhibition reached on once-a-day dosage is due to a balance being struck between inhibition only of active, acid-secreting pumps and de novo synthesis of new pumps or removal of omeprazole from inhibited pumps. Therefore, in order to obtain greater inhibition of secretion, it is more effective to increase dose frequency than dose quantity. This is discussed with respect to treatment of disease in Section IV.

It is inappropriate to combine simultaneous H_2 receptor antagonist therapy with omeprazole therapy, since the H_2 antagonist–dependent reduction in the number of active pumps will tend to reduce the efficacy of omeprazole. The H_2 receptor antagonist will add nothing in terms of therapeutic results.

Acid rebound does not seem to occur in man. Following omeprazole treatment, there is down-regulation of, or no change in, the level of the ATPase (36). In addition, the acid secretion returns to maximum only after about 96 hr in man, so that for the first few days after stopping treatment acid secretion remains below the level found before treatment.

Moreover, since the H^+,K^+-ATPase is the final step of acid secretion, it is not possible to develop tolerance to omeprazole, in contrast to the currently available H_2 receptor antagonists (9).

There is only one other site known where the gene for the gastric H^+,K^+-ATPase is expressed, and that is the cortical collecting duct of the kidney (39). The function of the pump in this region is not known, but it is present in extremely low levels, and acidity in this region does not reach the level necessary for accumulation of omeprazole.

◼ Consequences of Secretory Inhibition

It appears clear that maintained high acidity within the stomach is not required for health. In spite of many warnings to the contrary, acid suppression as a means of controlling ulcer disease has proved to be safe and without significant side effects.

Suppression of acid secretion by anti-secretory therapy, either with H_2 antagonists or pump inhibitors, results in elevated plasma gastrin levels (24,25). This follows from the decrease of the feedback regulation of gastrin release by intragastric pH, as described in Section II. The effect of pump inhibitor treatment on plasma gastrin levels in man is illustrated in figures 31A and B. Hypergastrinemia can have two major effects which can alter the efficacy of anti-secretory agents: increased histamine release and hyperplasia of parietal and ECL cells.

The elevated gastrin levels stimulate the ECL cells to release additional histamine, which in turn has the potential to produce a more intense stimulation of the parietal cell. With increased release of histamine, H_2 receptor antagonists may become less effective, and this may lead to secretory breakthrough during treatment. Up-regulation of alternative stimulatory pathways, such as vagal stimulation of muscarinic receptors or direct gastrin stimulation of the parietal cell, may also induce tolerance for receptor antagonists. Tolerance is found, for example, with treatment by the H_2 receptor antagonists after 2 weeks, probably reducing their efficacy by more than 50%. Increased doses of ranitidine did not appear to reverse the tolerance, suggesting that alternative pathways of acid secretory stimulation had been up-regulated and that tolerance is not due to changes in the levels of the H_2 receptor itself (9). Since the pump inhibitors act independently of the intensity or pathway of stimulus, tolerance is seen with this class of anti-secretory agent. The effect of elevated serum gastrin is stimulation of pump activity by the release of histamine.

Increasing the number of active pumps increases the efficacy of omeprazole; thus, this physiological effect improves the pharmacological response to omeprazole. A comparison of H_2 receptor antagonist properties and those of omeprazole is shown in figure 32.

In rats, long-term treatment with effective anti-secretory agents is associated with hypergastrinemia and often selective hyperplasia of the ECL cells (26–30). This increase of serum gastrin for all clinically used agents is due to the continuation of stimulation of gastrin release from the G-cell by food in the absence of the brake placed on gastrin release by the presence of acid in the antrum. Similar effects on ECL cells have been obtained after corpectomy or after gastrin infusion in the rat, (31,32). The effect of inhibition of acid secretion on ECL cell density disappears after antrectomy, which removes gastrin from the circulation. The ECL cell hyperplasia in rats therefore depends on the elevation of plasma gastrin induced by inhibition of acid secretion. In rats, the gastrin levels are about 10-fold greater than in humans after secretory inhibition. ECL hyperplasia is found to progress in the rat over a two-year treatment period with anti-secretory drugs, to assemblages of the ECL cells in the rats which are called carcinoids (33). In humans, long-term treatment with omeprazole over a period of 7 years has not been shown to result in ECL cell carcinoid formation or in drug-related ECL cell hyperplasia (24,25,34). The slight increase found in some patients in the number of ECL cells has been ascribed to a progression in atrophic gastritis rather than to a progression of ECL numbers (34). The ECL cell in the rat appears to have a particular sensitivity to serum gastrin levels. Not only is this heightened sensitivity of the ECL cell to gastrin absent in man, but secretory inhibition in people does not result in the same degree of elevation of serum gastrin (figures 31A and B).

Recent studies using isolated rat enterochromaffin-like cells have shown that gastrin alone, in the absence of any additional growth factors, is able to stimulate ECL cell DNA synthesis in vitro and that omeprazole, lansoprazole, and pantoprazole are without effect on DNA synthesis by the ECL cell (35). Hence, there appear to be no

(text continues on p. 90)

FIG. 31A. The effect of omeprazole treatment on gastrin levels in man as compared to highly selective vagotomy and untreated controls. It can be seen that although omeprazole elevates serum gastrin, it does so less than vagotomy. The elevation in pernicious anemia is much greater than the maximum elevation shown here.

FIG. 31B. The effect of long-term treatment of patients with omeprazole on serum gastrin. There is an initial elevation over the first 3 months of therapy and then there is no further change even after 4 years of treatment.

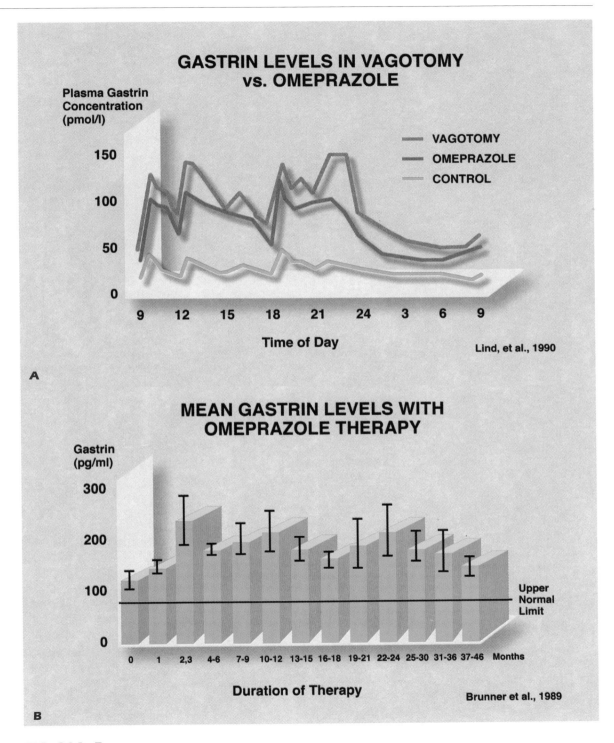

FIG. 31A, B

FIG. 32. A comparison of the properties and efficacy of H_2 receptor antagonists and acid pump inhibitors. Many effects are similar, but the molecular mechanism of action distinguishes omeprazole in terms of its efficacy and spectrum of action. Presented in this comparison are the relative merits of these two major types of drugs used in the treatment of acid-related diseases. It can be seen that pH control, treatment results, duration of action, dosing convenience, onset of action, lack of tolerance, and lack of acid rebound favor the use of acid pump inhibition in all approved indications.

H2 RECEPTOR ANTAGONISTS
VS.
ACID PUMP INHIBITORS

SIMILARITIES

REVERSIBLE INHIBITION
OF ACID SECRETION

FEW SIDE EFFECTS

FEW ADVERSE REACTIONS

HYPERGASTRINEMIA

EFFECTIVE IN DU, GU

DIFFERENCES

MOLECULAR TARGET

EFFICACY AND DURATION
OF ACTION

EFFECTIVE IN GERD II-IV

* EFFECTIVE WITH SINGLE
ANTIBIOTIC IN H. PYLORI
ERADICATION

*EFFECTIVE IN NSAID ULCERS

* UNDER INVESTIGATION

FIG. 32

direct effects of the drug on the ECL cell, and the observed ECL cell hyperplasia is due to the elevation of plasma gastrin levels induced by the inhibition of acid secretion. This hypergastrinemia occurs as a physiological, not pharmacological, response to all forms of secretory inhibition including vagotomy and H_2 receptor antagonists.

■ Comparative Pharmacology

The two classes of anti-secretory agents, H_2 receptor antagonists and acid pump inhibitors, share many properties, as listed in figure 32. They both reversibly inhibit acid secretion, have few side effects, and are effective, but not equally so, in peptic ulcer and reflux disease. The H_2 antagonists differ among themselves largely in terms of potency, not efficacy. Interactions with other drugs exist experimentally, but this is rarely of clinical consequence. Both classes of agents elevate serum gastrin, but not to levels that are of clinical significance.

The differences noted between the substituted benzimidazoles and the H_2 antagonists result from the difference in molecular target and chemical mechanism of action. The H_2 receptor antagonists are designed to inhibit only that part of acid secretion that depends on stimulation of the H_2 receptor. Since omeprazole binds to the acid pump, it is able to inhibit acid secretion irrespective of stimulus. The plasma half life of the available H_2 receptor antagonists is relatively short and hence their duration of action is also short. Since omeprazole binds covalently to the acid pump it has a long duration of action in spite of a short plasma half life. This consequence of its mechanism of action has resulted in significant therapeutic benefits as compared to the receptor antagonists in gastroesophageal reflux disease, duodenal ulcer, and Zollinger-Ellison syndrome with respect to both healing rates and symptom relief.

REFERENCES

1. Herzog P., Grendahl T., Linden J., Schmitt K.F., and Holtermueller, K.H.: Adverse effects of high dose antacid regimen, Results of a randomized, double-blind trial. Gastroenterology 80, 1173, 1980.
2. Feldman, M.: Inhibition of gastric acid secretion by selective and nonselective anticholinergics. Gastroenterology 86, 361, 1984.
3. Jaup, B.H., and Bloomstrand, C. H.: Cerebro-spinal fluid concentration of pirenzepine after therapeutic dosage. Scand. J. Gastroenterol. 15, 35, 1980.
4. Black, J. W., Duncan W. A. M., Durant, C. J., Ganellin, C. R., and Parsons, M. E.: Definition and antagonism of histamine H_2 receptors. Nature 236, 385, 1972.
5. Brimblecombe, R. W., Duncan, W. A. M., Durant, G. J., Emmett, J. C., Ganellin, C. R., Leslie, G. B., and Parsons, M. E.: Characterization and development of cimetidine as a histamine H_2-receptor antagonist. Gastroenterology 74, 339, 1978.
6. Bertaccini, G., and Coruzzi, G.: Control of gastric acid secretion by histamine H_2 receptor antagonists and anticholinergics. Pharmacol. Res. 21, 339, 1989.
7. Carter, D. C., Forrest, J., Werner, W., Heading, R. C., Park, J., and Shearman, D. J. C.: Effect of histamine H_2-receptor blockade on vagally induced gastric acid secretion in man. Br. Med. J. 3, 554, 1974.

8. Feldman, M., and Burton, M. E.: Histamine H_2 receptor antagonists. N. Engl. J. Med. 323, 1672, 1990.

9. Nwokolo C.U., Smith J.T. Gavey, C., Sawyer, A. and Pounder, R.E.: Tolerance during 29 days of conventional dosing with cimetidine, nizatidine, famotidine or ranitidine. Aliment. Pharmacol. Ther. 4 Suppl 1 p29-45, 1990.

10. Forte, T. M., Machen, T. E., and Forte, J. G.: Ultrastructural changes in oxyntic cells associated with secretory function. A membrane recycling hypothesis. Gastroenterology 73, 941, 1977.

11. Feldman, M., and Burton, M. E.: Histamine H_2 receptor antagonists. Part two. N. Engl. J. Med. 323, 1749, 1990.

12. Sachs, G., Chang, H. H., Rabon, E., Schackman, R., Lewin, M., Saccomani, G.: A non-electrogenic H^+ pump in plasma membranes of hog stomach. J. Biol. Chem. 251, 7690, 1976.

13. Ganser, A. L. and Forte, J.G.: K^+-stimulated ATPase in purified microsomes of bullfrog oxyntic cells. Biochim. Biophys. Acta 307, 169, 1973.

14. Fellenius, E., Berglindh, T., Sachs, G., Olbe, L., Elander, B., Sjostrand, S. E., and Wallmark, B.: Substituted benzimidazoles inhibit gastric acid secretion by blocking H/K-ATPase. Nature 290, 159, 1981.

15. Lorentzon, P., Jackson, R., Wallmark, B., and Sachs, G.: Inhibition of $(H^+ +K^+)$-ATPase by omeprazole in isolated gastric vesicles requires proton transport. Biochim. Biophys. Acta 897, 41, 1987.

16. Lindberg, P., Nordberg, P., Alminger, T., Brandstrom, A. and Wallmark, B.: The mechanism of action of the gastric acid secretion inhibitor omeprazole. J. Med. Chem. 29, 1327, 1986.

17. Sachs, G., Carlsson, E., Lindberg, P., and Wallmark, B.: Gastric H/K-ATPase as therapeutic target. Ann. Rev. Pharmacol. Toxicol. 28, 269, 1988.

18. Besancon, M., Shin, J. M., Mercier, F., Munson, K., Miller, M., Hersey, S. J., and Sachs, G.: Membrane topology and omeprazole labelling of the gastric H^+,K^+-Adenosinetriphosphatase. Biochemistry 32, 2345, 1993.

19. Scott, D. R., Helander, H. F., Hersey, S. J., and Sachs, G.: The site of acid secretion in the mammalian parietal cell. Biochim. Biophys. Acta 1146, 73, 1993.

20. Sachs, G., J. M. Shin, M. Besancon, and Prinz, C.: The continuing development of gastric acid pump inhibitors. Aliment. Pharmacol. Ther. 7(Suppl1): 4, 1993.

21. Shin, J. M. S., Besancon, M., Simon, A., and Sachs, G.: The site of pantoprazole in the gastric H^+K^+-ATPase. Biochim. Biophys. Acta 1148, 223, 1993.

22. Regårdh, C.-G., Gabrielsson, M., Hoffman, K.-L., Löfberg, I., and Skånberg, I.: Pharmacokinetics and metabolism of omeprazole in animals and man—an overview. Scand. J. Gastroenterol. 20, 79, 1985.

23. Lind, T., Cederberg, C., Ekenved, G., Haglund, U., and Olbe, L.: Effect of omeprazole—a gastric acid pump inhibitor—on pentagastrin stimulated acid secretion in man. Gut 24, 270, 1983.

24. Brunner, G. H. G., Lamberts, R., and Creutzfeld, W.: Efficacy and safety of omeprazole in the long-term treatment of peptic ulcer and reflux oesophagitis resistant to ranitidine. Digestion 47(Suppl 1):64, 1990.

25. Kohn, A., Annibale, B., Prantera, C., Giglio, L., Suriano, G., and Delle-Fave, G.: Reversible sustained increase of gastrin and gastric acid secretion in a subgroup of duodenal ulcer patients on long term treatment with H_2 antagonists. J. Clin. Gastroenterol. 134, 284, 1991.

26. Larsson, H., Carlsson, E., Mattson, H., Lundell, L., Sundler, F., Sundell, G., Wallmark, B., Watanabe, T., and Hakanson, R.: Plasma gastrin concentrations and gastric enterochromaffin-like cell activation and proliferation. Gastroenterology 90, 391, 1986.

27. Ryberg, B., Tielemanns, Y., Axelson, J., Carlsson, E., Hakanson, R., Mattsson, H., Sundler, F., and Willems, G.: Gastrin stimulates the self-replication of enterochromaffin-like cells in the rat stomach. Gastroenterology 99, 935, 1990.

28. Tielemanns, Y., Hakanson, R., Sundler, F., and Willems, G.: Proliferation of enterochromaffin-like cells in omeprazole treated hypergastrinemic rats. Gastroenterology 96, 723, 1989.

29. Wallmark, B., Skaenberg, I., Mattson, H., Andersson, K., Sundler, F., Hakanson, R., and Carlsson, E.: Effects of 20 weeks ranitidine treatment on plasma gastrin levels and gastric enterochromaffin-like cell density in the rat. Digestion 45, 181, 1990.

30. Tielemanns, Y., Axelson, J., Sundler, F., Willems, G., and Hakanson, R.: Serum gastrin affects the self-replication rate of enterochromaffin-like cells in the rat stomach. Gut 31, 274, 1990.

31. Mattson, H., Havu, N., Braeutigam, J, Carlsson, K., Lundell, L., and Carlsson, E.: Partial gastric corpectomy results in hypergastrinemia and development of gastric enterochromaffin-like carcinoids in the rat. Gastroenterology 100, 311, 1991.

32. Ryberg, B., Axelson, J., Hakanson, R., Sundler, F., and Mattson, H.: Trophic effects of continuous infusion of [Leu15]-gastrin-17 in the rat. Gastroenterology 98, 33, 1990.

33. Havu, N.: Enterochromaffin-like cell carcinoids of the gastric mucosa after life-long inhibition of gastric secretion. Digestion 35, 42, 1986.

34. Lamberts, R., Creutzfeldt, W., Strueber, H. G., Brunner, G., and Solcia, E.: Long-term omeprazole therapy in peptic ulcer disease, Gastrin, endocrine cell growth, and gastritis. Gastroenterology 104, 1356, 1993.

35. Prinz, C., Scott, D. R., Hurwitz D, Helander H.F. and Sachs, G.: Gastrin effects on isolated rat enterochromaffin-like cells in primary culture. Amer. J. Physiol. 267, G663, 1994.

36. Scott D., Besancon M., Sachs, G. and Helander H.F.: The effect of antisecretory drugs on parietal cell structure and H+,K+-ATPase levels in rabbit gastric mucosa in vivo. Dig Dis Sci 39, 2118, 1994

37. Nwokolo C.U., Smith J.T., Sawyerr A.M. and Pounder R.E.:Rebound intragastric hyperacidity after abrupt withdrawal of histamine H$_2$ receptor blockade. Gut 32, 1455, 1991

38. Besancon M. and Sachs G.: The critical cysteine for omeprazole inhibition of the gastric ATPase. Gastroenterology 1995 in press

39. Kraut, J.A., Birmingham S., Sachs, G. and Reuben M.A.: The presence of the gastric H,K ATPase in renal tissue. Amer. J. Physio.l 1995 in press.

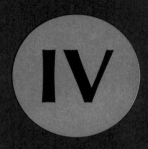

IV

Management of Acid-Related Disorders

OVERVIEW

Patients presenting in a doctor's office with upper gastrointestinal symptoms range from those with vague complaints and distress, usually classified as non-ulcer dyspepsia, to those in whom a specific disease can be diagnosed by objective criteria. Gastritis, or inflammatory infiltration of the wall of the stomach, may account in part for non-ulcer dyspeptic symptoms. These patients are a diagnostic and therapeutic challenge. The diagnosis of an acid-related disease such as esophagitis or gastric or duodenal ulcer can be often established based on symptoms and history alone. The therapeutic approach involves a choice of different means of acid suppression for acute treatment of these diseases, and effectiveness of therapy often confirms the diagnosis. In the case of gastric ulcer, it is important to exclude gastric neoplasia as contributory to the symptoms, best done by endoscopic biopsy. Following acute treatment, relapse must be a consideration in treatment. Prevention of relapse involves either symptomatic discontinuous therapy or maintenance treatment with anti-secretory drugs.

Many diseases of the upper gastrointestinal tract are dependent on the presence of gastric acid. Either the organ is exposed abnormally to acid or responds abnormally to acid. The most frequently presenting of these are gastroesophageal reflux disease, duodenal ulcer, and gastric ulcer. Current medical management of these disorders is based on the general therapeutic goal of reducing gastric acidity. The acid-related disorders differ in terms of pathogenesis and sensitivity to gastric acid levels. Therefore, different levels and duration of acid secretory suppression are required for optimal healing and symptomatic relief in the different diseases. In other words, there are targets for the degree and duration of acid secretory suppression required for optimal healing of acid-related disease. If the target pH elevation and duration is reached, healing and symptom relief are optimized.

In the case of esophagitis, agents have been developed that increase the tone of the esophageal sphincter. These agents, however, are not specific for this particular region of smooth muscle, and initial clinical data indicate lower efficacy than agents that suppress acid secretion.

Extensive clinical trials have been performed to evaluate the efficacy of the two classes of the most popular anti-secretory agents, H_2 receptor antagonists and the acid pump inhibitor omeprazole. Both classes provide significant therapeutic benefit for healing and symptomatic relief of uncomplicated disorders. On a relative basis, omeprazole is found to have significant therapeutic advantage over the H_2 antagonists in terms of the rate and percentage success of healing. This is particularly evident with erosive reflux esophagitis and duodenal ulcer. This therapeutic advantage is related to the more effective and more sustained suppression of acid secretion obtained with acid pump inhibition. Over 90 million treatments have been performed world-wide using omeprazole and 4 million with lansoprazole. Pantoprazole is in the process of registering in different countries. No side effects and few adverse events have been noted, showing that this class of drug is well tolerated and safe. In clinical trials, the compounds have shown similar efficacy and similar profiles in different treatment areas. Another PPI, E3810, 2-(4-methyl-3-methoxypropoxy)pyridyl-methylsulfinyl-benzimidazole is entering phase III trials, even though it is significantly less stable at neutral pH than any of the other compounds.

Recently, there has been increasing awareness of the role of *Helicobacter pylori* in peptic ulcer recurrence. A recent consensus meeting at the National Institutes of Health has recommended eradication of *H. pylori* concomitant with anti-secretory therapy. For eradication the possibilities listed were triple therapy, omeprazole therapy with antibiotic and perhaps an H_2 antagonist with two antibiotics (27). Only the last two regimens combine anti-secretory therapy with eradication. Of these, treatment with omeprazole and antibiotic is necessary for 2 weeks, and the combination with H_2 receptor antagonists is necessary for 2 weeks, with an additional 4 to 6 weeks of treatment for healing.

Figures illustrating this section are figures 33 through 37.

THERAPEUTIC GOALS

The goal of therapy in this category of disease is to provide rapid healing and rapid symptomatic relief, avoid complications, and prevent recurrence. To date, this goal has been best achieved by inhibition of acid secretion by the stomach, but the increasing awareness of the need to eradicate *H. pylori* is holding out the promise of a cure for duodenal and gastric ulcers.

All of the acid-related disorders respond positively to suppression of gastric acid secretion. However, the extent to which gastric pH must be elevated in order to obtain optimal symptomatic relief and healing is different for treatment of reflux esophagitis or peptic ulcers, as illustrated in figure 33. These differences probably relate to the etiology of the disorders.

Control of acid secretion as it relates to healing rates in duodenal ulcer and reflux esophagitis has been quantified using meta-analysis of a large number (almost 300) of double-blind clinical trials (reviewed in refs. 1–4). In the meta-analysis, healing rates were compared to the expected 24-hour values of intragastric acidity using pH metry, and curves were constructed to determine the level of pH and the duration at that level required to achieve optimal healing rates (5,6).

For treatment of duodenal ulcer the meta-analysis indicates that if a target pH of 3 is achieved for at least 16–18 hours out of a 24-hour period, the maximal healing rate is achieved and no further improvement is expected with further elevation of intragastric pH or longer duration at the target pH. In the case of reflux esophagitis, optimal healing requires a target pH of 4 for 16 out of the 24 hours (5,6). Again, no improvement is anticipated with greater pH elevation or duration of increased pH. Thus greater acid inhibition is required for treatment of esophagitis than for duodenal ulcer disease. In evaluating intragastric pH as a prediction of treatment results, it should not be forgotten that it is probably the acid load on the duodenum that determines disease, and that it is gastric wall pH which determines whether *H. pylori* is eradicated with a single antibiotic in combination with a proton pump inhibitor.

A preliminary analysis has been performed to define the target pH for eradication of the bacterium *H. pylori* using only a single antibiotic such as amoxicillin.

FIG. 33. *A diagram showing the optimal pH levels and the duration for which these pH levels have to be maintained for optimal healing of duodenal ulcer and esophagitis, based on a meta-analysis of double-blind clinical trials. It can be seen that these desired pH levels are well achieved by omeprazole on once-a-day dosing, less so by ranitidine on twice-a-day dosing. Further inhibition of acid secretion has no further healing effects in these diseases as illustrated by the meta-analyses. (From Hunt and his colleagues, refs. 5,6).*

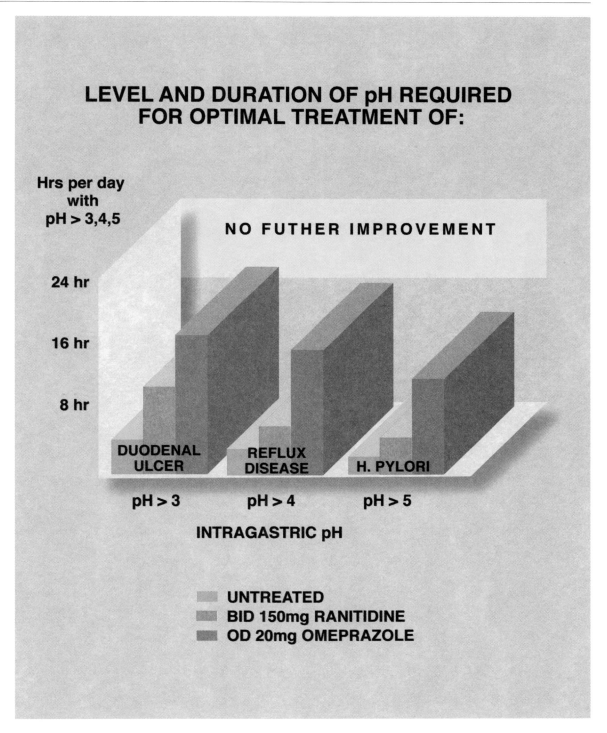

LEVEL AND DURATION OF pH REQUIRED FOR OPTIMAL TREATMENT OF:

Hrs per day with pH > 3,4,5

NO FUTHER IMPROVEMENT

24 hr

16 hr

8 hr

DUODENAL ULCER   REFLUX DISEASE   H. PYLORI

pH > 3   pH > 4   pH > 5

INTRAGASTRIC pH

- UNTREATED
- BID 150mg RANITIDINE
- OD 20mg OMEPRAZOLE

FIG. 33

This analysis is included because of the strong association of this bacterium with duodenal ulcer. Current clinical trials are aimed at evaluating eradication protocols with the objective of preventing relapse and even curing ulcer disease. For eradication of *H. pylori* with a single antibiotic the target intragastric pH is probably 5, perhaps for 24 hours a day. This goal requires even more profound inhibition than for the treatment of esophagitis (7). It should be pointed out that luminal pH does not reflect wall pH accurately, certainly at low rates of acid secretion where neutralization in the lumen elevates pH much above that of the wall. The acid pump transports 160 mM HCl, with appropriate volume flow. So 90% inhibition of pumps will result in acid production within the gastric wall at 10% volume, and the acidity will still be very high. In the lumen, since HCO_3^- secretory capacity is 10% of acid secretory capacity, much of this 10% residual secretion may be neutralized, but not within the gastric wall itself. These factors are of importance when considering the results of gastric ulcer therapy and results of trials designed to eradicate *H. pylori*.

In summary, the results of this type of analysis show that H_2 receptor antagonists fail to achieve the target pH for a sufficient period of time to provide optimal healing in duodenal ulcer and fall far short of the target pH for erosive reflux esophagitis (stage II–IV). Once-a-day (20 mg) omeprazole achieves the target pH for sufficient time to provide optimal healing in duodenal ulcer. This dose is able also to achieve optimal healing in the majority of patients with erosive esophagitis.

Thus when considering a target pH for 75–80% of the day for any acid-related disease as well as for eradication of *H. pylori* with growth-dependent antibiotics, only omeprazole and similar compounds are able to achieve this target at reasonable dose. In order to understand the dose–acid inhibition relationship, it is necessary to consider the pharmacodynamics of omeprazole and other PPI's.

PHARMACODYNAMICS OF OMEPRAZOLE AND OTHER PPI'S

The PPI class of drug is virtually unique in therapy in that a covalent binding occurs to the target molecule, the H^+,K^+-ATPase. It might be thought that this would instantaneously inhibit acid secretion for a long time. However, this is not so. Firstly, the drugs have a short plasma half-life, about 60 minutes following oral dosing, and less following acute IV administration. Secondly, the drugs are active only against functional pumps, and not all pumps are working at the same time. To ensure that pumps are being stimulated, one should take the drug just before meals, such as, for example, one half-hour before breakfast. Night-time dosing, when the majority of pumps are inactive, is not recommended, in contrast to H_2 receptor antagonists. As long as the plasma levels and pump activation coincide, acid secretion will be switched off. Since probably not all pumps can be activated simultaneously, some pumps will escape the first dose of drug.

In the ensuing 24 hours, a fraction of the pumps will be replaced by de novo synthesis. The half-life of pump protein in the rat is 50 hr (48), but recovery of acid secretion or ATPase activity after omeprazole inhibition is considerably faster, being about 19 hr (49). Omeprazole does not alter the rate of turnover of pump protein, so this must mean that in the rat some pumps reactivate. In man, the effective half-life of omeprazole inhibition is 48 hr. This may be due also to a combination of synthesis and recovery of inhibited pumps. Hence, in patients, about 25% of pumps renew or reactivate every 24 hr (50,51).

We do not know the percentage of active pumps at breakfast, when omeprazole is given, but a reasonable assumption is that about 75% of the pumps present in the parietal cell are active during exposure to the drug. Hence, with the first dose, about 75% are inhibited, and 25% acid secretory capacity remains following the dose. Over the next 24 hr, this secretory capacity remains and 25% of pumps renew or are made, to give a total secretory capacity 24 hr after first dose of 50%. With the second dose, 75% of these will be inhibited, leaving a secretory capacity of 12% following this second dose. Again during the day, 25% of pumps reappear, to give a secretory capacity of 37% prior to the third dose. With inhibition of 75% of these pumps, 9% capacity remains, to be joined again by 25% pump capacity appearing during the next 24 hr to give 34% capacity available prior to the fourth dose. So with repeated single daily dosing on the average about 30% of secretory capacity re-appears in man prior to the next dose, as indeed has been found (50). These calculations are illustrated in figure 34. Twice-a-day dosage will improve the pH profile and has been found sometimes beneficial in Zollinger-Ellison syndrome and in people with particularly severe reflux.

It must be remembered, however, that the final acid secretory capacity calculations reflect what is available in terms of secretory capacity the next morning just before the next dose, and that the recovery of acid secretion is gradual throughout the 24 hr following dose. Thus after the second dose, only 11% of original pump capacity is available, most of which will be neutralized by either food or HCO_3^- secretion, until night-time, when a low-volume, high-acidity juice is produced. It can be seen therefore that once-a-day dosing will result in an elevation of pH >3 for 75% of the day even after the second dose of omeprazole or other pump inhibitors.

If it is necessary to abolish acid secretion, for example in order to neutralize the fundic area to promote growth of *H. pylori*, this once-a-day regimen will be inadequate and more frequent dosing of omeprazole will be required. What these considerations also illustrate is the possible basis for attacking different targets with antibiotics for elimination of *H. pylori*. Growth-dependent targeting obtains in these regions where organisms are growing, such as the antrum. Here amoxicillin will be effective, being an antibiotic that depends on bacterial division for its action. In the fundus, which is much more acid, no or little growth will occur and metronidazole is necessary for killing the organism in the stationary state, since metronidazole does not require cell replication for its action. Clarithromycin, which inhibits bacterial protein synthesis, is only partially growth-dependent and may turn out to be the most effective antibiotic in combination with proton pump inhibitors.

The synergism between omeprazole and amoxicillin and other similar types of antibiotics probably lies in the fact that, by elevation of pH, omeprazole stimulates growth of the bacteria in the fundus as well as the antrum. Thus the organism will become sensitive to amoxicillin not only in the antrum but in the fundus as well. It is reasonable to suggest that for reliable eradication of *H. pylori* with a single antibiotic in combination with omeprazole, the dose of omeprazole will have to be increased in frequency so that true abolition of acid secretory capacity is extended for five days. This is the usual duration of treatment for antibacterial therapy with amoxicillin and similar antibiotics.

(text continues on p. 102)

FIG. 34. Illustration of the pharmacodynamics of acid inhibition and pH elevation by omeprazole.

The figure is a three-dimensional plot illustrating the pump capacity immediately before the first or subsequent doses of a pump inhibitor (before drug), the pump capacity immediately after the drug has taken effect (after drug), and the percentage of time the intragastric pH is greater than 3.0.

The first row shows that 100% of pump capacity is present before the first dose. 75% of these pumps are active during the presence of the drug and are therefore inhibited, leaving 25% pump capacity immediately after the first dose (second row). With an effective half life of 48 hr, 25% of pumps are synthesized or recover during the first day, giving about 50% pump capacity prior to second dose, as shown in the first row. Again 75% of these are inhibited, giving, immediately after the second dose, about 12% pump capacity remaining (as shown in the second row). Again, new pumps are synthesized or some pumps recover, to give about 37% pump capacity immediately before the third dose. 9% remains after this dose. In the last row, the % of time expected for the pH to be greater than 3 is shown. Since the pump recovery continues throughout the day, and is assumed to be uniform, even after the first day, only 37% average capacity returns, giving significant inhibition of intragastric acidity even on the first day. With the second dose, average pump capacity is reduced to 25% but most returns in the evening, when stimulation of secretion is minimal. Given neutralization by food and bicarbonate secretion, it can bc calculated that the intragastric pH should be elevated above 3 for about 60% of the day even with the second dose. Steady-state inhibition reaches 70% of pump capacity immediately before the next dose, leaving a residual 7% following dose, sufficient to elevate intragastric pH to the optimal level for healing of duodenal ulcers (5,6, and unpublished observations).

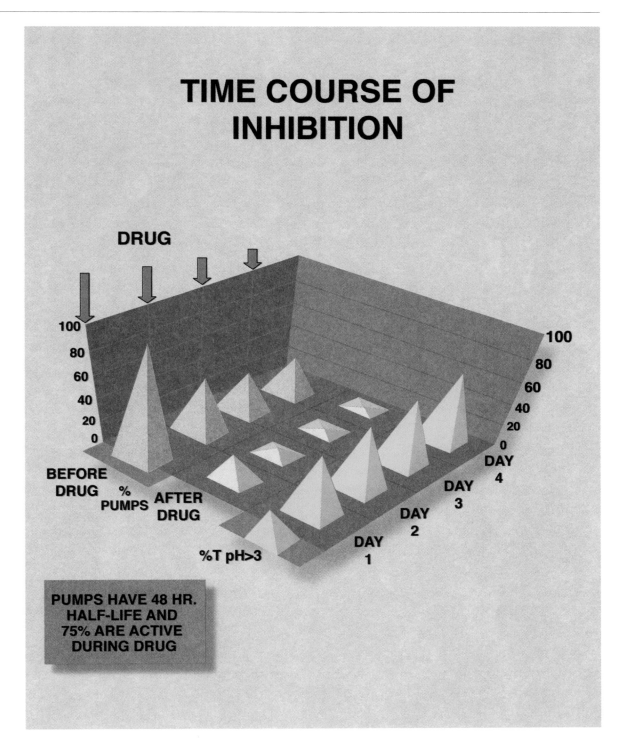

FIG. 34

MANAGEMENT STRATEGY

Gastroesophageal Reflux Disease

Reflux esophagitis is a common disease resulting from prolonged exposure of the distal esophagus to acidic gastric contents, usually due to incompetence of the esophageal sphincter. Heartburn, acid regurgitation, and dysphagia are the major symptoms. Twenty four hour esophageal pH monitoring is a non-invasive test for determining that the esophagitis is due to reflux. Endoscopy is used to confirm the diagnosis and to classify the stage of this disease.

Reflux esophagitis is divided endoscopically into four stages, according to severity of the mucosal lesions. The clinical spectrum of the uncomplicated disease ranges from reflux symptoms without evidence of esophageal damage (stage 0) to erosive and ulcerative esophagitis (stage II–IV).

Since the most important factor in the pathophysiology of reflux esophagitis is the abnormal exposure of the esophageal mucosa to acid, anti-secretory therapy has a major beneficial effect. Inhibition of gastric acid secretion is the most frequently used therapeutic approach in this disease. Prokinetic agents such as cisapride, designed to constrict the esophageal sphincter, are less often used, mainly because it has been difficult to design a drug selective for the lower esophageal sphincter that is also as effective as pump inhibition. Surgical procedures on the lower esophagus, such as fundoplication, remain another option in the young patient able to tolerate surgery.

The optimum acid inhibitory regimen for reflux esophagitis requires a sustained intragastric pH above 4 for between 16 and 18 hr per day (5). This treatment goal is more easily attained with acid pump inhibition than with H_2 antagonists, as shown in figure 33.

Although H_2 receptor antagonists at standard doses provide symptom relief for some patients, it is appears that these are relatively ineffective at providing complete symptom resolution and healing in most patients with stage II to IV erosive esophagitis. This is likely because of the failure of H_2 receptor antagonists to reduce intragastric acidity to the level required for optimal healing rates and symptom resolution. For this reason, higher and more frequent doses of H_2 receptor antagonists must be given, with the caveat of tolerance and acid rebound. For example, the ranitidine label was changed to four-times-a-day dosing for patients with erosive esophagitis.

Placebo-controlled clinical trials (8,9) have shown good endoscopic healing rates (81%) with omeprazole after 4 weeks (vs. 6% with placebo), and 75% of patients were symptom free (e.g. heartburn), demonstrating the efficacy of omeprazole in both healing and symptom relief. Several randomized multicenter studies (10-17) have shown that omeprazole has a significant therapeutic advantage over treatment with standard doses of ranitidine or cimetidine in healing erosive and ulcerative lesions and relieving symptoms in patients with reflux esophagitis. Esophagitis healed in 56–81% of patients after four weeks of omeprazole therapy, and in 71–96% after eight weeks, while H_2 receptor antagonists had a healing rate of 26–39% at 4 weeks and 23–66% at 8 weeks. The relative lack of efficacy of the lower doses of ranitidine led to recommendation of a higher dosage frequency, but as yet there has not been a comparison between omeprazole and 150 mg ranitidine given 4 times a day, the dose currently approved for treatment by this drug in the United States. Figure 35 illustrates that omeprazole is the drug of choice for stage II and higher GERD.

Relapses in patients with reflux esophagitis are frequent and occur early, up to 60% within 3 months, 82% after 6 months when no treatment is given (18). These patients often require long term treatment to prevent further relapses. In overseas studies, continuous maintenance (17,18) therapy with omeprazole (20mg/ day) over 1 year showed remission rates of 78-89% to be compared to 25-38% with H_2 receptor antagonists. Omeprazole is not yet approved for maintenance use in the United States but protocols with omeprazole are under investigation.

It does not seem that infection with *H. pylori* is causal for reflux disease. Eradication therapy for *H. pylori* is therefore unlikely to provide additional benefit in this acid-related disease.

■ Duodenal Ulcer

Duodenal ulcers present as an acute or chronic disease of the proximal duodenum in which there is a lesion of the mucosa which may penetrate to the submucosa and beyond. The symptoms are diffuse and vary among individuals, but epigastric pain, especially during the night, with pain relief after antacid or meal ingestion is the most common symptom reported. Increased incidence of duodenal ulcers has been shown in smokers, young males (incidence up to 5% of the population), and patients taking non-steroidal anti-inflammatory medication such as aspirin. Complications such as bleeding or perforation are common, and the presence of tarry stools may be the first sign of the disease.

Duodenal ulcer disease is associated, in almost every case, with chronic antral gastritis and *H. pylori* infection. This epidemiological association suggests strongly that the presence of this bacterium is critical in the pathogenesis of duodenal ulcer disease. Duodenal ulcers have never been reported to mask underlying malignancies, in contrast to gastric ulcers, and therefore do not require extensive biopsy.

The inhibition of gastric acid secretion by H_2 receptor antagonists has become the standard approach to management in both acute and maintenance therapy for duodenal ulcers since the introduction of this class of drug. Four H_2 receptor antagonists (cimetidine, ranitidine, famotidine, and nizatidine) have been approved in the United States for this treatment. Following treatment with H_2 receptor antagonists, healing rates for duodenal ulcer are reported as 51, 78, and 92% after 2, 4, or 8 weeks of treatment at the recommended doses (4). Treatment is improved significantly by pump inhibition with omeprazole, as shown in figure 36.

The efficacy of omeprazole in the treatment of duodenal ulcers was first demonstrated in non-comparative, placebo-controlled studies (19–22). At once-a-day dosing, omeprazole achieved complete healing of duodenal ulcer in 61–83% of patients after 2 weeks and in 91–100% after 4 weeks.

Numerous multicenter double-blind studies have subsequently compared the efficacy of omeprazole to the efficacy of H_2 receptor antagonists in the management of duodenal ulcers. Overall, omeprazole (20 mg once a day) provided faster symptomatic relief and faster duodenal ulcer healing than with H_2 receptor antagonists such as cimetidine, ranitidine, or famotidine (23–33). After two weeks of treatment, ulcers healed in 42–83% of the patients treated with omeprazole and in 34–63% with ranitidine treatment. Statistical meta-analysis (1) showed a significant therapeutic gain for omeprazole of as much as 30% in the first two-week treatment. After four weeks, ulcers in the omeprazole (20 mg/day)-treated group healed in 82–97% of the patients.

Higher doses (40 mg/day) of omeprazole have been shown to provide additional benefit when risk factors are present. Risk factors that might require the higher dose or longer treatment period include poor response to H_2 receptor antagonists, large ulcer size (>10 mm), smoking, and early onset of the disease (before age 30). In five open studies in patients responding poorly to H_2 receptor antagonist treatment, 40 mg of omeprazole over 4–8 weeks produced healing in 98% of the patients (1,2).

Relapse rates of duodenal ulcers are frequent, 83% after 12 months. Thus prevention of relapse is important in management of duodenal ulcer disease. One approach to management of relapse is maintenance therapy with H_2 receptor antagonists. Another is symptomatic treatment, but ulceration may occur without symptoms.

Comparative foreign studies focused on relapse have shown similar remission rates after stopping treatment with H_2 receptor antagonists or omeprazole (34,35). Following acute treatment with omeprazole (10–20 mg/day), the relapse rate was between 59 and 71% after 6 months, and following acute ranitidine treatment (300 mg/day) the relapse rate was 54% after 6 months and 88% after 12 months. Under maintenance therapy using H_2 receptor antagonists, the relapse rate drops to about 16% (45). Similar decreases of relapse rates have been obtained with omeprazole (20). A new, promising approach that is being intensively investigated is eradication of *H. pylori*, as discussed below.

It has been shown that eradication of *H. pylori* reduces the frequency of ulcer relapse (46). This suggests that future treatment of duodenal ulcer disease may well involve both acid suppression and *H. pylori* eradication, the idea being to cure the disease. If these epidemiological data hold true, maintenance therapy for virtually all patients with duodenal ulcer disease will no longer be required provided that there is effective and permanent eradication of *H. pylori* along with anti-secretory therapy. As can be seen, the concept that *H. pylori* together with acid secretion is an essential factor in duodenal ulcer disease has revised our understanding of the pathogenesis of duodenal ulcer disease. At the time of writing this review, we would anticipate that eradication of this organism at the time of treatment of the acid-related disease would possibly cure duodenal ulcer disease in most patients.

(text continues on p. 108)

FIG. 35. A schematic diagram for treatment of erosive esophagitis (grade II–IV), showing the symptoms, diagnosis, treatment options and therapeutic gain comparing omeprazole and H_2 antagonists.

REFLUX DISEASE

SYMPTOMS
HEARTBURN, DYSPHAGIA, REGURGITATION

DIAGNOSIS
ENDOSCOPY, CLASSIFICATION 0, I-IV

TREATMENT
EROSIVE TO ULCERATIVE

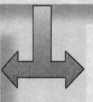

H2 RECEPTOR ANTAGONISTS

RANITIDINE (ZANTAC) 150 mg QID
FAMOTIDINE (PEPCID) 40 mg BID
NIZATIDINE (AXID) 150 mg BID

8-12 WEEKS

OMEPRAZOLE (PRILOSEC)

20-40 mg/OD

4-8 WEEKS

THERAPEUTIC GAIN IN COMPLETE HEALING AND SYMPTOM RELIEF OF REFLUX ESOPHAGITIS

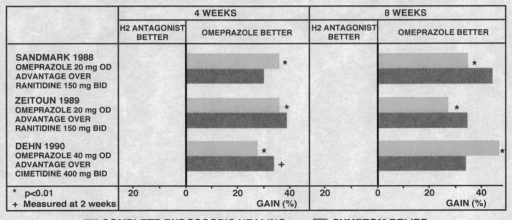

FIG. 35

FIG. 36. A schematic diagram for treatment of duodenal ulcer, showing the symptoms, diagnosis, treatment options and therapeutic gain comparing omeprazole and H$_2$ antagonists.

DUODENAL ULCER DISEASE

SYMPTOMS
EPIGASTRIC PAIN, MEAL OR ANTACID RELIEF

DIAGNOSIS
ENDOSCOPY, X-RAY

TREATMENT

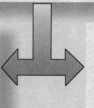

H2 RECEPTOR ANTAGONISTS
RANITIDINE (ZANTAC) 300 mg HS
CIMETIDINE (TAGAMET) 300 mg HS
FAMOTIDINE (PEPCID) 40 mg HS
NIZATIDINE (AXID) 300 mg HS
4-8 WEEKS

OMEPRAZOLE (PRILOSEC)
20 mg/OD

2-4 WEEKS

THERAPEUTIC GAIN IN DUODENAL ULCER HEALING AT TWO AND FOUR WEEKS

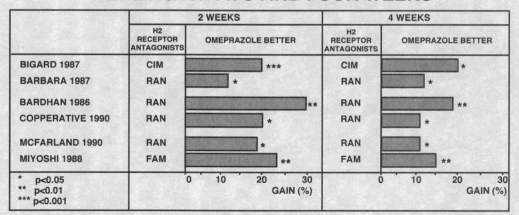

* p<0.05
** p<0.01
*** p<0.001

CIM = CIMETIDINE 400mg BID vs. OMEPRAZOLE 20mg OD
RAN = RANITIDINE 150mg BID vs. OMEPRAZOLE 20mg OD
FAM = FAMOTIDINE 20mg BID vs. OMEPRAZOLE 20mg OD

FIG. 36

■ Gastric Ulcer

The etiology of gastric ulcers appears similar to that of duodenal ulcers. In both disorders the formation of lesions depends on the presence of acid aided by peptic activity in the gastric juice. Epidemiological studies have also implicated *H. pylori* infection in a large fraction of gastric ulcer patients (46). In addition, the use of non-steroidal anti-inflammatory drugs (NSAID's) such as aspirin contributes significantly to the occurrence of gastric ulcers that are not related to *H. pylori* infection. High steroid use, especially in infants, results in gastric ulceration, and it is often seen in intensive care units. In contrast to duodenal ulcer patients, patients with gastric ulcers are rarely hypersecretors. The most frequent site of gastric ulceration is at the antral/fundic junction. A reasonable explanation for the lack of correlation of intragastric pH and the occurrence of gastric ulceration is that it is the pH within the gastric wall which determines the acid dependence of gastric ulcers, not the pH at the surface of the mucosa. For this pH to be elevated to close to neutrality, essentially all acid secretion must be inhibited.

Clinically, endoscopy is necessary to establish the diagnosis, and several tissue specimens need to be examined histologically to exclude a possible underlying malignancy. Gastric ulcers are found primarily in the lesser curvature of the stomach, and any other location is suspicious for malignancy.

Standard therapy for this disease has been the administration of ranitidine or cimetidine. Healing rates of gastric ulcers above 80% using a therapy with H_2 receptor antagonists have required treatment over 8–12 weeks (4). The requirement for long treatment duration may be explained in part by the persistence of a low intramural pH even though the intragastric pH is elevated by this therapy to a level above 3.

This discrepancy in pH between gastric wall and gastric lumen is due to neutralization of the secreted acid after it has left the gastric epithelium, but not before. Because the acid pump secretes 160 mM HCl if it is working at all, even a few functioning pumps will acidify the gastric wall. Therefore a more effective inhibition of acid secretion is expected to be a superior means of management in the treatment of gastric ulcers. It seems, however, that the degree of acid inhibition necessary for optimization of gastric ulcer healing may have been underestimated.

FIG. 37. A schematic diagram for treatment of gastric ulcer, showing the symptoms, diagnosis and treatment options.

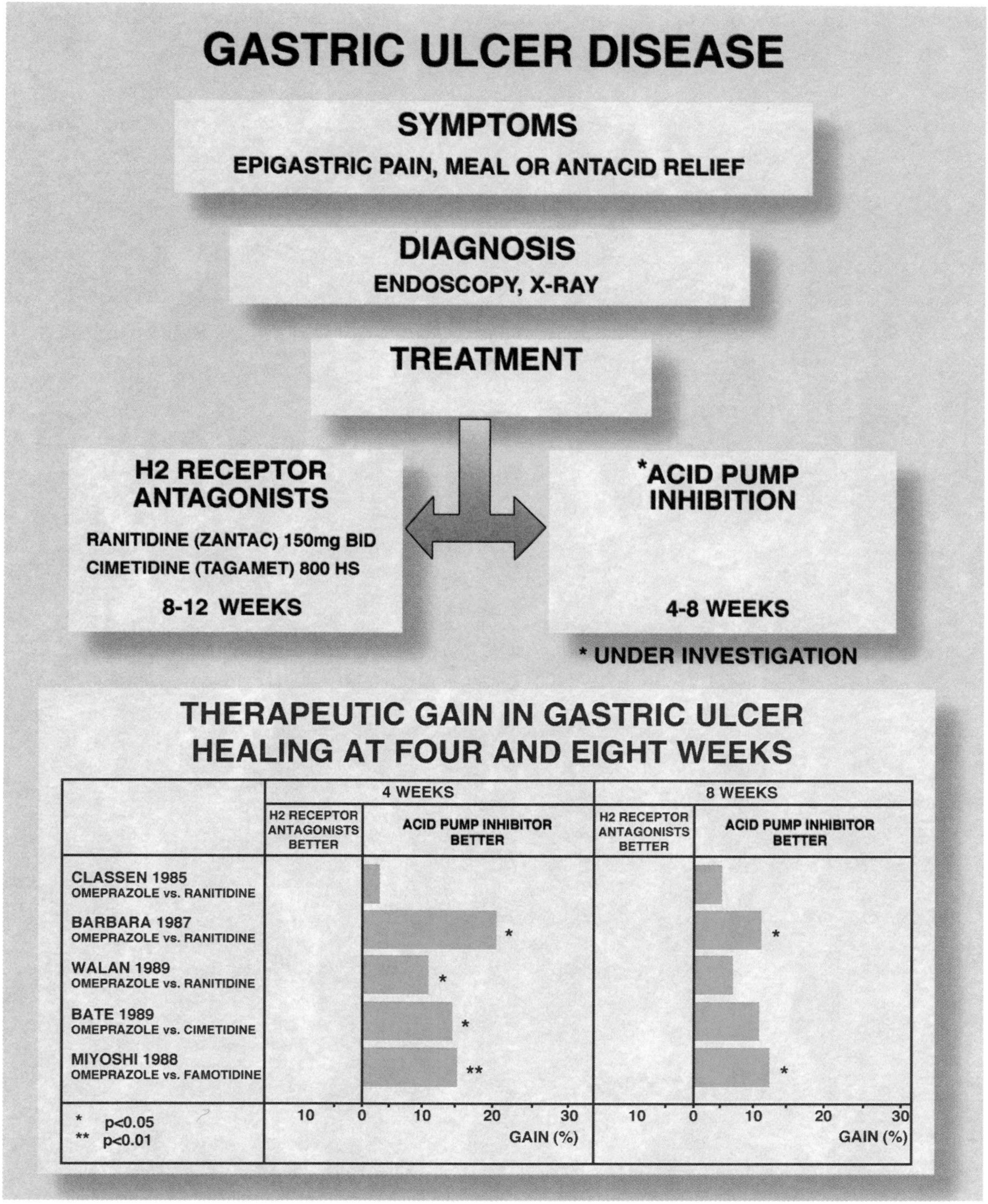

GASTRIC ULCER DISEASE

SYMPTOMS
EPIGASTRIC PAIN, MEAL OR ANTACID RELIEF

DIAGNOSIS
ENDOSCOPY, X-RAY

TREATMENT

H2 RECEPTOR ANTAGONISTS

RANITIDINE (ZANTAC) 150mg BID

CIMETIDINE (TAGAMET) 800 HS

8-12 WEEKS

*ACID PUMP INHIBITION

4-8 WEEKS

* UNDER INVESTIGATION

THERAPEUTIC GAIN IN GASTRIC ULCER HEALING AT FOUR AND EIGHT WEEKS

	4 WEEKS		8 WEEKS	
	H2 RECEPTOR ANTAGONISTS BETTER	ACID PUMP INHIBITOR BETTER	H2 RECEPTOR ANTAGONISTS BETTER	ACID PUMP INHIBITOR BETTER
CLASSEN 1985 OMEPRAZOLE vs. RANITIDINE				
BARBARA 1987 OMEPRAZOLE vs. RANITIDINE		*		*
WALAN 1989 OMEPRAZOLE vs. RANITIDINE		*		
BATE 1989 OMEPRAZOLE vs. CIMETIDINE		*		
MIYOSHI 1988 OMEPRAZOLE vs. FAMOTIDINE		**		*

* $p < 0.05$
** $p < 0.01$

10   0   10   20   30
GAIN (%)

10   0   10   20   30
GAIN (%)

FIG. 37

Most studies have shown superiority of acid pump inhibition when compared to H_2 receptor antagonists (39-41), as shown in figure 37. Non-comparative studies (36-38) have shown that omeprazole administered once daily healed gastric ulcers in 70–72% of patients after 4 weeks. Further, several randomized comparative multi-center studies (24,35,39,40,41) have compared omeprazole with H_2 receptor antagonists in patients with gastric ulcers. Where 20 mg omeprazole once a day was used, healing rates were 59–74% after 4 weeks. After 8 weeks, ulcers healed in 85–96% of patients. Symptomatic relief with omeprazole treatment was achieved after 2 weeks and antacid consumption decreased by 65% after the first 3 weeks of treatment.

Among patients with gastric ulcers responding poorly to H_2 receptor antagonist treatment, therapy with omeprazole 40 mg/day for 8 weeks resulted in 92–100% healing (39).

The smaller advantage on behalf of the acid pump inhibitors relative to H_2 receptor antagonists in the treatment of gastric ulcers as compared to erosive esophagitis or duodenal ulcer may be due to the fact that the omeprazole was only given at standard dosage once per day, which may not be the optimal dosage for ulcers in this region. Thus, when 40 mg od omeprazole was administered, 80% healing was achieved at 4 weeks and improved further at 8 weeks (35). This study may indicate that higher or divided doses of acid pump inhibitors might be necessary to decrease the intramural pH sufficiently for optimal healing rates in gastric ulcer disease.

Relapse of gastric ulcers is relatively frequent (45% one year after stopping antisecretory therapy). The current treatment strategy to prevent recurrence is maintenance therapy with cimetidine or ranitidine, similar to the treatment of duodenal ulcers, although therapy with acid pump inhibitors may replace current H_2 antagonist therapy in the near future. Currently, several new treatments are being evaluated in the patients with frequent relapse (3 relapses in 2 years). These now include triple antibiotic therapy along with an antisecretory agent or a combined treatment with acid pump inhibitor and single antibiotics such as amoxicillin or clarithromycin for *H. pylori* eradication.

It is often the case that gastric ulceration is caused by the use of NSAID's, and a careful history must be taken to determine if the patient is using this class of drug. In fact, most, if not all cases of gastric ulceration resistant to acid pump inhibitors have turned out to be due to excessive NSAID consumption.

The role of *H. pylori* in gastric ulceration appears significant also. Current opinion holds that *H. pylori* infection is necessary for gastric ulcer disease unless the patient is taking NSAID's (46). As eradication protocols are being investigated, more data should become available linking *H. pylori* infection to the etiology of gastric ulcer disease.

■ Zollinger-Ellison Syndrome

Zollinger-Ellison syndrome is a rare disease due to gastrin cell tumors characterized by extreme hypersecretion of gastric acid and intractable ulceration. The symptoms are due to the excessive gastric acid secretion stimulated by the gastrin secreted from the causative gastrinoma. To determine the long-term efficacy and safety of omeprazole in the management of this disease, an extensive prospective long-term study has been performed in 40 patients for 6–51 months (42). The mean daily dose of omeprazole was 82 mg. Omeprazole healed the ulcers and prevented mucosal lesions in all patients including 17 patients previously non-responsive to H_2 receptor antagonists. No significant side effects were observed, and serum gastrin concentrations did not change significantly. Similar results were also found in less extensive studies (43,44). For these reasons omeprazole should be the drug of choice for treatment of this disease. Interestingly, *H. pylori* is absent in these patients, presumably due to the very high acidity in the stomach.

REFERENCES

1. Maton, PN.: Omeprazole. N. Engl. J. Med. 324, 965, 1991.

2. McTavish, D., Buckley, M. M. T., and Heel, R. C.: Omeprazole. An updated review of its pharmacology and therapeutic use in acid-related disorders. Drugs 42, 138, 1991.

3. Feldman, M., and Burton, M. E.: Histamine H2 receptor antagonists. N. Engl. J. Med. 323, 1672, 1990.

4. Feldman, M., and Burton, M. E.: Histamine H2 receptor antagonists. Part two. N. Engl. J. Med. 323, 1749, 1990.

5. Bell, N. J. V., Burget, D., Howden, C. W., Wilkinson, J., and Hunt, R. H.: Appropriate acid suppression for the management of gastroesophageal reflux disease. Digestion 51, 59, 1992.

6. Burget, D.W., Chiverton, S.G., and Hunt, R.H.: Is there an optimal degree of acid suppression for healing of duodenal ulcers? Gastroenterology 99, 345, 1990.

7. Chiba N., Rao B.V., Rademaker J.W., and Hunt R.H.: Meta-analysis of the efficacy of antibiotic therapy in eradicating H. Pylori. Am. J. Gastroenterol. 87, 1716, 1992.

8. Dent, J.: Australian clinical trials of omeprazole in the management of reflux esophagitis. Digestion 47, 69, 1990.

9. Hirschowitz, B. I., Holt, S., Robinson, M., Behar, J., Sontag, S., et al.: Omeprazole is superior to placebo in the complete relief of heartburn and endoscopic healing in patients with reflux esophagitis, US multicenter dose ranging study results. Abstract. Am. J. Gastroenterol. 84, 1144, 1989.

10. Bate, C. M., Keeling, P. W. N., O'Morain, C. A., Wilkinson, S. P., Mountford, R. A., et al.: Omeprazole provides faster healing and symptom relief of reflux esophagitis than cimetidine. Gut 30, A1493, 1989.

11. Dehn, T. C. B., Shepherd, H. A., Colin-Jones, D., Kettlewell, M. G. W., and Carrol, N. G. H.: Double-blind comparison of omeprazole (40mg od) versus cimetidine (400mg qd) in the treatment of symptomatic erosive reflux esophagitis, assessed endoscopically, histologically, and by 24h pH monitoring. Gut 31, 509, 1990.

12. Havelund, T., Laursen, L. S., Skoubo-Kristensen, E., Andersen, B. N., Pedersen, S. A., et al.: Omeprazole and ranitidine in the treatment of reflux esophagitis, double-blind comparative trial. Br. Med. J. 296, 89, 1988.

13. Lundell, L., Backman, L., Ekstrom, P., Enander, L. K., Fausa, O., et al.: Omeprazole or high-dose ranitidine in the treatment of patients with reflux esophagitis not responding to standard doses of H2 receptor antagonists. Aliment. Pharmacol. Ther. 4, 145, 1990.

14. Sandmark, S., Carlsson, R., Fausa, O., and Lundell, L.: Omeprazole or ranitidine in the treatment of reflux esophagitis. Scand. J. Gastroenterol. 23, 625, 1988.

15. Vantrappen, G., Rutgeerts, L., Schurmans, P., and Coenegrachts, J.-L.: Omeprazole (40 mg) is superior to ranitidine in short term treatment of ulcerative reflux esophagitis. Dig. Dis. Sci. 33, 523, 1988.

16. Zeitoun, P., Rampal, P., Barbier, P., Isal, J. P., Eriksson, S., et al.: Omeprazole (20mg) versus ranitidine (150mg bid) in reflux esophagitis. Gastroenterol. Clin. Biol. 13, 457, 1989.

17. Dent, J., Klinkenberg-Knol, E. C., Elm, G., Eriksson, K., Rikner, L., et al.: Omeprazole in the long term management of reflux esophagitis refractory to histamine H2 antagonists. Scand. J. Gastroenterol. 24, 176, 1989.

18. Hetzel, D. J., Dent, J., Reed, W. D., Narielvala, F. M., and MacKinnon, M.: Healing and relapse of severe peptic esophagitis after treatment with omeprazole. Gastroenterology 95, 903, 1988.

19. Bader, J. P., Modigliani, R., Soule, J. C., Delchier, J. C., Morin, R., et al.: An open trial of omeprazole in short-term treatment of duodenal ulcer. Scand. J. Gastroenterol. 21, 177, 1986.

20. Cooperative Study Group, Omeprazole in duodenal ulceration, acid inhibition, symptom relief, endoscopic healing, and recurrence. Br. Med. J. 289, 525, 1984.

21. Karvonen, A. L., Keyrilainen, O., Uusitalo, A., Salaspuro, M., Tarpila, S., et al.: Effects of omeprazole in duodenal ulcer patients. Scand. J. Gastroenterol. 21, 419, 1986.

22. Scandinavian Multicenter Study. Gastric acid secretion and duodenal ulcer healing during treatment with omeprazole. Scand. J. Gastroenterol. 19, 882, 1984.

23. Barbara, L., Blasi, A., Cheli, R., Corinaldesi, R., Dobrilla, G., et al.: Omeprazole vs ranitidine in the short term treatment of duodenal ulcer, an Italian multicenter study. Scand. J. Gastroenterol. 21, 177, 1986.

24. Bardhan, K. D., Naesdal, J., Bianchi Porro, G., Petrillo, M., Lazzaroni M., et al.: Treatment of refractory peptic ulcer with omeprazole or continued H2 receptor antagonists, a controlled clinical trial. Gut 32, 435, 1991.

25. Delle Fave, G., Annibale, B., Helander, H., Puoti, M., Corleto, V., et al.: Omeprazole versus high dose ranitidine in H2 blocker resistant duodenal ulcer patients. Eur. J. Gastroenterol. and Hepatol. 3, 337, 1991.

26. Gloria, V. I., Domingo, E. O., Makalinao, A. U., Zano, F. M., Rasco, E. T., et al.: A comparison of omeprazole and ranitidine in the management of patients with duodenal ulcer. Eur. J. Gastroenterol. Hepatol. 3, 215, 1991.

27. McFarland, R. J., Baetson, M. C., Green, J. R. B., O'Donoghue, D. P., Dronfield, M. W., et al.: Omeprazole provides quicker symptom relief and duodenal ulcer healing than ranitidine. Gastroenterology 98, 278, 1990.

28. Mulder, C. J. J., and Schipper, D. L.: Omeprazole and ranitidine in duodenal ulcer healing. Analysis of comparative clinical trials. Scand. J. Gastroenterol. 25, 62, 1990.

29. Sabbatini, F., Piai, G., and Mazzacc, G.: Italian multicentre studies with omeprazole in the treatment of peptic ulcer disease. Ital. J. Gastroenterol. 20, 20, 1988.

30. Valenzuela, J. E., Berlin, R. G., Snape, W. J., Johnson, T. J., Hirschowitz, B. I., et al.: US experience with omeprazole in duodenal ulcer. Multicenter double-blind comparative study with ranitidine. Dig. Dis. Sci. 36, 523, 1988.

31. Bigard, M. A., Isal, J. P., Galmiche, J. P., Ebrard, F., Bader, J. P., et al.: Omeprazole versus cimetidine in short term treatment of acute duodenal ulcer. Gastroenterol. Clin. Biol. 11, 753, 1987.

32. Hetzel, D. J., Korman, M. G., Hansky, J., Eaves, E. R., Shearman, D. J. C., et al.: A double blind multicentre comparison of omeprazole and cimetidine in treatment of duodenal ulcer. Aust. N. Z. J. Med. 16, 595, 1986.

33. Miyoshi, A., et al.: The effect of omeprazole and famotidine on duodenal ulcer—a double blind comparative study. Jap. Pharmacol. Ther.. 16, 563, 1988.

34. Lauritsen, K., Andersson, B. N., Laursen, L. S., Hansen, J., Havelund, T., et al.: Omeprazole 20 mg three days a week and 10 mg daily in prevention of duodenal ulcer relapse. Gastroenterology 100, 663, 1991.

35. Walan, A., Bader, J. P., Classen, M., Lamers, B. H. W., Piper, D. W., et al.: Effect of omeprazole and ranitidine on ulcer healing and relapse rates in patients with benign gastric ulcer. N. Engl. J. Med. 320, 69, 1989.

36. Farup. P. G., Darle, N., Falk, A., and Bernklev, T.: Treatment of benign gastric ulcer with omeprazole 30 mg once daily. Cur. Ther. Res. 43, 872, 1988.

37. Francavilla, A., Ingrosso, M., Mogelli, A., Baldassare, M., Giaccari, S., et al.: Omeprazole, a new anti-secretory drug in the treatment of gastric ulcer. Dig. Dis. Sci. 31, A335, 1986.

38. Huttemann, W.: Short term treatment of gastric ulcer with once daily omeprazole. Scand. J. Gastroenterol. 21, 179, 1986.

39. Brunner, G., and Creutzfeldt, W.: Omeprazole in the long-term management of patients with acid-related diseases resistant to ranitidine. Scand. J. Gastroenterol. 24, 101, 1989.

40. Cooperative Study Group.: Double blind comparative study of omeprazole and ranitidine in patients with duodenal or gastric ulcer, a multicenter trial. Gut 31, 653, 1990.

41. Bate, C. M., Wilkinson, S. P., Bradby, G. V. H., Bateson, M. C., Hislop, W. S., et al.: Randomized, double-blind comparison of omeprazole and cimetidine in the treatment of gastric ulcer. Gut 30, 1323, 1989.

42. Maton, P. N., Vinayek, R., Frucht, H., McArthur, K. A., Miller, L. S., et al.: Long-term efficacy and safety of omeprazole in patients with Zollinger Ellison syndrome. A prospective study. Gastroenterology 97, 827, 1989.

43. Cadranel, J. F., Ruszniewski, P., Elovaer-Blanc, L., Lehy, T., Delchier, J. C., et al.: Long term efficacy and tolerability of omeprazole in 20 patients presenting severe Zollinger Ellison syndrome. Gastroenterol. Clin. Biol. 13, 654, 1989.

44. Hirschowitz, B. I., Deren, J., Raufman, J. P., Lamont, B., Berman, R., et al.: A US multicenter study of omeprazole treatment of Zollinger-Ellison syndrome. Gastroenterology 94, 595, 1988.

45. Holtmann G, Armstrong D, Blum A L, Arnold R, Classen M, Goebell H, Fischer M.: Effects of 2 year maintenance therapy with ranitidine on the natural course of duodenal ulcer disease. Gastroenterology 102, A84, 1992

46. Malfertheimer P., Ditschuneit et al.: Helicobacter pylori, gastritis, and peptic ulcer. Springer Verlag, Berlin, Germany 1990,

47. Unge, P., Olsson, J., Gad, A., and Gnarpe, H.: Does omeprazole, 40 mg om, improve antimicrobial therapy directed towards gastric Campylobacter pylori in patients with antral gastritis? Scand. J. Gastroenterol. 24(Suppl. 166):184, 1989.

48. Gedda, K., D. Scott, M. Besancon, and G. Sachs.: The half life of the H,K ATPase of gastric mucosa. Gastroenterology 106, A79, 1994.

49. Wallmark, B., H. Larsson, and L. Humble.: The relationship between gastric acid secretion and gastric H^+, K^+-ATPase activity. J. Biol. Chem. 260, 13681, 1985.

50. Von Muller P, Seite HK, Simon B et al.: Vierwochige Omeprazole Gabe, Einfluss auf Saeureverhalten und basale Hormonspiegel. Z. Gastroenterolog. , 22, 236 ,1984.

51. Naesdal, J., Bodemar, G. and Walan A.: Effect of omeprazole, a substituted benzimidazole, on 24 hr intragastric acidity in patients with peptic ulcer disease. Scand. J. Gastroenterol. 19, 916 , 1984.

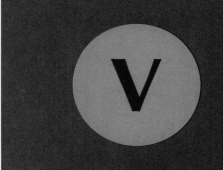
Future Trends

OVERVIEW

The previous sections of this book have dealt with the mechanism and control of acid secretion in relation to healing peptic ulcer disease and reflux esophagitis. At the present time, control of acid secretion is the best approach available not only for treating these diseases, but also for providing rapid and effective symptom relief. Despite all of the advances that have been made in understanding gastric physiology, biochemistry and molecular biology, the precise etiology of duodenal and gastric ulcer remains unclear. Esophagitis is thought to result from acid reflux into the lower esophagus due to incompetence of the lower esophageal sphincter. In the case of Zollinger Ellison syndrome, it is the hyperacidity due to the constant stimulation by gastrin that determines the presence of ulceration. With the advent of the proton pump inhibitor drugs, we now have as an effective means of control of acid secretion as is necessary, superior in all respects to the histamine-2 receptor antagonists. The next task for research in this area is to develop knowledge about *H. pylori*, its biology, its toxicology and appropriate means for its eradication.

As our understanding of the scientific basis of acid secretion has become more sophisticated, medical therapy has replaced dietetic or surgical therapy. We can anticipate continuing progress in medical treatment of peptic ulcer disease as a result of improved knowledge in two general areas, the etiology of ulcer disease and the mechanisms of epithelial regeneration. Both are complicated problems. A contributory cause of duodenal and gastric ulcer disease is the presence of *H. pylori* in the stomach. Epithelial regeneration involves interplay between a variety of cytokines and adhesion factors, largely undefined in the gastrointestinal tract. As etiology and regeneration become better defined, improvements in therapy will follow.

Figure 38 through 40 relate to this section.

■ Etiology of Ulcer Disease

Peptic ulcer disease is caused by inappropriate destruction of the gastric and duodenal epithelium. Acid is required for this destruction to occur. For acid to have injurious effects on the epithelium, it has to be able to penetrate below the surface of the epithelium. The presence of acid in the interstitial space has the potential to lower intracellular pH to levels incompatible with cell survival. Acid injury is likely exacerbated by the presence of peptic activity beneath the surface of the epithelium. There are various mechanisms whereby the gastric epithelium resists acid.

Most importantly, the apical cell membrane, which is normally exposed to the high acidity found in the stomach, is acid-impermeable (1). The cells are joined close to their apex by tight junctions which also are essentially acid-impermeable (2). In addition, the surface cells, but not the peptic cells, which are also exposed to acid, secrete mucus and partially neutralize the acid by means of bicarbonate secretion (3).

It is unlikely that disease changes the permeability of the apical membrane to acid. However, when chemicals such as aspirin are added which can transport acid across plasma membranes, the acid-permeability is drastically increased (4). This effect of NSAID's explains, in part, the frequent occurrence of NSAID-induced gastric ulcer disease. The inhibition of prostaglandin biosynthesis by these agents is probably also related to their ulcerative action.

However, it is possible to conceive of disease or infection altering the permeability of the tight junctions. If this is increased, acid penetrates to the basal-lateral surface of the gastric epithelium. This surface is permeable to protons. Hence, if enough acid penetrates after disruption of the tight junctions, gastric mucosal damage will result from intracellular acidification. It is also thought that the acid environment that then exists within the tissue maintains peptic activity, which adds to the damage being caused by the acid itself by hydrolyzing basement membrane, collagen and even blood vessel walls. This concept is illustrated in figure 38.

It appears that the presence of a bacterium, *Helicobacter pylori*, is closely associated with the occurrence of duodenal and non-NSAID gastric ulcers in the population (5,6). Perhaps infection with this organism is required before tight junctions are disrupted. A tight junction between oxyntic cells is illustrated in figures 39A and 39B. Acid would then be able to penetrate the epithelium and ulcer disease result. Further, the presence of *H. pylori* might contribute to non-ulcer dyspepsia, but additional studies have to be performed to evaluate the organism's role in this important group of symptoms.

Other factors beyond acid and *H. pylori* infection must also contribute to the occurrence of duodenal and gastric ulcers, since a large percentage of the population has both acid secretion and *H. pylori* infection present yet does not suffer from ulcer disease. Various factors have been invoked, such as local ischemia, inappropriate sites of acid secretion such as are found in Barrett's disease of the esophagus or foci of gastric metaplasia in the duodenum, but none of these are as yet established as primary causes. As research progresses on the interaction of *H. pylori* and the gastric mucosa, these factors will be clarified.

In contrast to duodenal and gastric ulcers, reflux disease is thought to be due mainly to incompetence of the lower esophageal sphincter, with consequent acid damage to the lower esophagus. There are several prokinetic drugs (e.g., metoclo-

(text continues on p. 122)

FIG. 38. A conceptual model of the development of ulcer disease, showing a progressive disruption of tight junctions, with acid back diffusion, progressive cell damage, and eventual cell death and massive acid entry. The initiation of tight junction disruption is postulated to relate to infection with *H. pylori*.

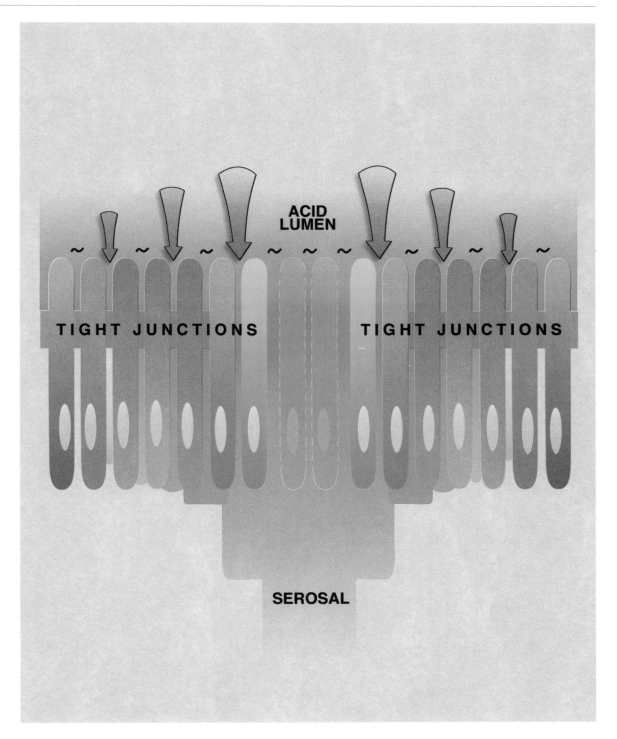

FIG. 38

FIG. 39A. An illustration of a tight junction at the electron microscopic level, using lanthanum infiltration. It can be seen that lanthanum permeates between the basal lateral surface but not into the tight junctions.

FIG. 39B. A freeze fracture of a tight junction between oxyntic cells showing the large number of tight junction strands with protein particles preventing back diffusion of acid. The orientation of this micrograph is lumen above.

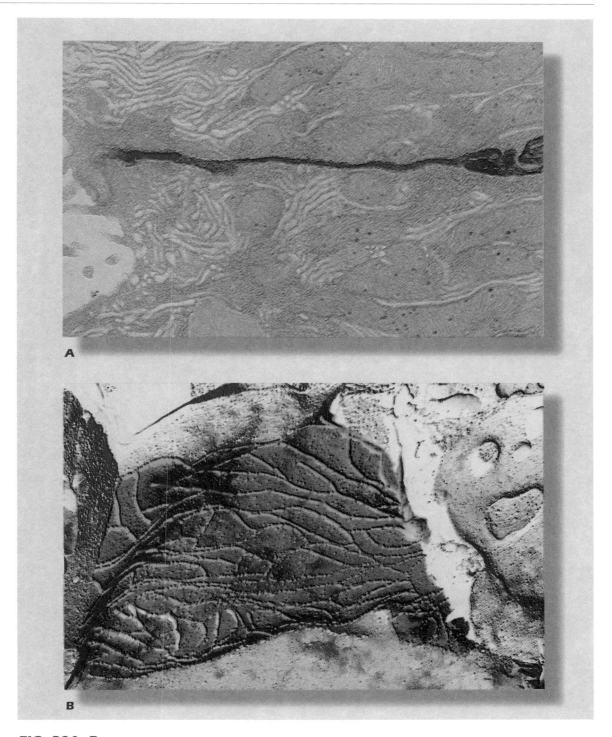

FIG. 39A, B

pramide or cisapride) available which enhance esophageal sphincter contraction. In general these have proven relatively ineffective in severe disease, but are therapeutically effective in mild reflux disease. Various factors may contribute to this therapeutic variation, such as absence of effect of the prokinetic agents on transient relaxation of the esophageal sphincter or the degree of incompetence of the sphincter. However, the understanding of smooth muscle contraction and its regulation is advancing rapidly, and newer drugs might be more effective than those available currently.

Inhibition of acid secretion to treat erosive esophagitis seems to require elevation of intragastric pH to 4 for most of the day (7). To date, only the substituted benzimidazole class of pump inhibitor such as omeprazole is able to achieve this goal reliably.

Other types of acid pump inhibitor are under active investigation. In contrast to the covalent substituted benzimidazole class, there are chemicals such as imidazopyridines or aryl quinolines that act as K^+ competitive inhibitors of the acid pump. These are predicted to be as effective as the substituted benzimidazoles in elevation of gastric pH, since they also inhibit the acid pump, but to have a duration of action dependent entirely on their plasma half-life as for the receptor antagonists. None are yet approved for clinical use but several have been studied in man and shown to be effective inhibitors of acid secretion.

■ Healing and Symptom Relief

Healing of ulcer disease involves several stages. First, there has to be restitution of the epithelium separating the luminal and serosal surfaces of the organ. Then there has to be effective re-epithelialization of the surface of the tissue. Finally, the inflammatory response to ulceration has to be reversed. These cellular events involve several factors, both local and general, that are slowly being unraveled. For example, one hypothesis for the beneficial effect of sucralfate is that this sulfated saccharide stabilizes the TGFα produced by the damaged epithelium, aiding the healing process even in the presence of acid (8).

It would appear likely that in the near future, treatment of acid-related diseases will combine anti-secretory therapy with drugs designed to eradicate *H. pylori*. Wound healing promoters will also be evaluated in these diseases.

What actually determines symptomatic relief is not fully understood. The more effectively acidity is decreased, the more rapid the symptomatic relief, as shown for example by the rapid action of antacids in relieving heartburn. Further, acid pump inhibition produces more rapid symptomatic relief than H_2 antagonists because of its more effective suppression of acid secretion. However, other factors also play a role, for example inflammation and inflammatory mediators.

A factor that should also be taken into consideration in treatment design is the site of the acidic pH. Inhibition of secretion such that intragastric pH is elevated to about pH 3 for 16–18 hr a day appears sufficient for optimal healing of duodenal ulcers (9). It should be remembered that the duodenum has significant acid-neutralizing capability, so that this degree of elevation appears sufficient, such that duodenal secretion of bicarbonate takes care of this level of acidity. In contrast, for gastroesophageal reflux disease (grade II-IV), the pH has to be elevated to about 4 for the same time period for optimal healing, suggesting that the esophageal epithelium has little if any acid-neutralizing capacity.

In the case of gastric ulceration, whether spontaneous or caused by NSAID-induced acid damage, even if the pH in the gastric lumen is 4, there is still very significant acidity in the wall of the stomach, since this is the primary site of acid secretion. The primary acidity may be very high although of low volume, allowing most of it to be neutralized before it reaches the gastric lumen. Here neither pH-metric analysis nor titration of acidity reveals the pH of the gastric wall. It may therefore be necessary in the future, for optimal treatment of gastric ulcers, to inhibit acid secretion more completely than even for erosive esophagitis, for example by divided doses of pump inhibitors or by timed-release medication.

In the special case of NSAID-induced ulcers, the NSAID's inhibit cyclooxygenase, which synthesizes prostaglandins from arachidonic acid, thus preventing the synthesis of prostaglandins. One therapeutic approach to NSAID ulcers has been to use EP_3 active prostaglandin analogs such as misoprostol to treat this particular form of gastric ulceration by replacing the prostaglandin (10). However, there are multiple prostaglandin receptor subtypes, and an EP_3 agonist may not be the optimal subtype for gastric protection. An NSAID such as aspirin also acts as a proton transporter across biological membranes. In the presence of luminal acid, the gastric surface epithelial cells will be acidified, and damaged directly by aspirin-mediated acid entry. Hence prostaglandin replacement therapy may not be as beneficial as acid inhibition for this type of NSAID-induced gastric damage.

■ Helicobacter pylori

(i) General aspects

In the last decade, it has been recognized that not only is gastric acid essential for duodenal ulcer, but that habitation of the gastric mucosa by an organism, *Helicobacter pylori*, appears also to be required for the recurrence and even occurrence, of duodenal ulcer (5,6), and for the occurrence of gastric ulcers that are not associated with the ingestion of non-steroidal anti-inflammatory drugs such as aspirin (4). This organism plays no role in the pathogenesis of erosive esophagitis.

In addition to being associated with ulcer disease, the presence of the organism is also associated with gastritis (11). In turn there is some evidence that gastritis is associated with an increased risk of gastric neoplasia (12). Non-ulcer dyspepsia may also be associated with this infection.

Two goals are likely to be set for the future medical treatment of duodenal and gastric ulcers. One is of course to heal the ulcer and provide symptomatic relief. The second will be to prevent recurrence by eradication of *H. pylori* and thereby cure peptic ulcer disease in most patients. As the therapeutic goal of *H. pylori* eradication is achieved by simple drug regimens, it is likely that eradication of the organism will become a therapeutic goal independent of the presence of ulcer disease. This is because gastritis per se may predispose to gastric cancer and *H. pylori* causes gastritis (12). As epidemiologic data accumulate, it may well be that all *H. pylori* infections will require eradication. Prevention of infection by oral vaccination may become another option.

Until something better is found, the combination of PPI and antibiotic is probably the regimen of choice for eradication, even in the absence of peptic ulcer disease.

The systematic development of eradication strategies requires hypotheses and testing of these hypotheses, just as the presence of a histamine-2 receptor target or the presence of a gastric acid pump target were also working hypotheses. What is required is an understanding of why the organism is in the stomach, what enables it to survive and which cellular process is an appropriate target for drug design.

This organism occupies a unique ecological niche in human biology, the acid environment of the stomach. *H. pylori* is a flagellate, spiral, Gram-negative bacterium that has a cell wall. It belongs to the Campylobacter family, with 90% genetic identity. However, it colonizes the gastric mucosa, being found in the mucus layer, in pyloric glands, often in the region of the tight junctions between surface epithelial cells, and occasionally even in the secretory canaliculus of the parietal cell. It also colonizes areas of gastric metaplasia (13). Apart from binding to gastric cells, it may be that there is a requirement for a certain acidity to optimize the environment of the bacterium and excessive acidity prevents its occurrence, since neither pernicious anemia patients nor those with Zollinger-Ellison syndrome suffer from the infection.

The pH of the human stomach averages about 1.4 over a 24-hr period. The actual pH at the gastric surface is controversial, some believing that it is able to be neutral most of the time (14). It seems likely that at some point significant acidity must be present at this surface and certainly is present within the gastric oxyntic gland lumen. This means that within the stomach *H. pylori* is exposed, at least on occasion, to an acid environment, which kills bacteria such as *E. coli*, but *H. pylori* is able to survive this hostile environment. *H. pylori* must therefore have acid defense mechanisms.

The best studied of these defense mechanisms is urease. The organism produces large amounts of urease, present either in the periplasmic space or on the outside surface of the bacterium. Presumably the urea concentration in the stomach reflects blood concentration, i.e., 1–3 mM. The NH_3 produced by this external urease is thought to protect the organism against the high acidity of the mucosa by reacting with H^+ to form NH_4^+ (for reviews see refs 13, 23). Urease-negative mutants are unable to colonize the stomach in animal models (15). On the other hand, inhibition of urease does not eradicate the organism. It appears that urease is required for the organism to establish itself in an acidic environment, but once present, it is no longer essential for survival everywhere in the stomach. This finding could reflect the different pH values in different parts of the stomach. In the fundus, urease would be essential for the organism's survival; in the antrum, where the pH is higher, urease might not be essential.

It appears therefore that the organism is a facultative acidophile, which means that it is able to elevate its cytoplasmic pH above that of its general environment in order to survive acidic pH. This does not necessarily mean that it has properties in terms of proton pumping similar to the classical acidophiles (16). It may simply be that by generation of NH_3 either with urea hydrolysis by urease or with deamination of glutamine or asparagine, for example, neutralization of the periplasmic space or the cytoplasm of the organism is achieved. Urea is not necessary for growth at neutral pH but seems important for growth at more acidic pH values.

The organism is very similar to *Campylobacter jejuni*, a neutrophile. Apparently its adaptation to the gastric environment has involved developing a battery of genes, the urease operon, in order to generate buffer allowing it to survive. It is not known whether in addition there have been changes in the inner membrane pumps to allow maintenance of a proton motive force at lower than usual ambient pH's, as is the case with obligate acidophiles such as *Thiobacillus acidophilus*.

(ii) Proton pump inhibition and eradication

Many antibiotics such as amoxicillin and clarithromycin depend on cell division for their efficacy as antibiotics. Amoxicillin is targeted at cell wall biosynthesis, clarithromycin inhibits protein synthesis. Efficacy of the latter antibiotic may be less growth-dependent than the former. Others such as metronidazole, which attacks DNA, do not. However, metronidazole, being a weak base, will be excluded from the interior of an organism where cytoplasmic pH is elevated above medium pH and will be less effective in an acidic environment. Hence to eradicate *H. pylori* in its habitat, two classes of antibiotic appear to be required, one to kill the growing bacteria, the other to kill the resting bacteria.

From in vitro growth data, it should be possible to convert all the *H. pylori* to growth phase if the gastric wall pH is elevated sufficiently. This is only possible with a pump inhibitor such as omeprazole. If this elevation of pH is properly achieved, an antibiotic such as amoxicillin or clarithromycin or a combination of these should be able to eradicate *H. pylori* within 5–7 days, the usual treatment period with this type of antibiotic. However, if we consider the pharmacodynamics of the interaction of omeprazole with the pump and the biology of the pump, as discussed above, uniform elevation to a wall pH of 5.0 or so is approached but not achieved routinely with even twice-a-day therapy. The idea that pump inhibition results in pH elevation so that *H. pylori* grows and becomes susceptible to eradication with amoxicillin is illustrated in figure 40.

There is sufficient synergism between omeprazole and either amoxicillin or clarithromycin such that reasonable eradication rates may be achieved with bid drugs in combination over a 2-week treatment period (17–20). Thus highly effective suppression of acid secretion combined with one or two antibiotics (21–23) is currently under investigation as a means of *H. pylori* eradication. This combination of eradication and anti-secretory therapy has the advantage that the ulcer itself is being healed and symptoms are being treated while *H. pylori* is being eradicated (21–23). A combination of this type will always be required for treatment of peptic ulcer disease.

The hypothesis that is being pursued in this type of study is that with adequate inhibition of gastric acidity, single or dual antibiotic therapy should reach 100% efficacy. If neutral pH could be achieved, a cell wall–targeted antibiotic such as amoxicillin should be effective on its own. Failing this, the addition of metronidazole to the regimen should take care of those bacteria still surviving in acid but not dividing.

There have been claims of a direct action of proton pump inhibitors on *H. pylori* at pH 7 in vitro, and extrapolation of this effect to the in vivo situation. It is quite unlikely that such a mechanism accounts for the synergism between antibiotics and proton pump inhibitors. Rather this in vitro effect reflects solution instability of the drugs, rather than any specific action. The explanation for the synergism and ineffectiveness of PPI's in vivo on their own is more likely related to pH elevation than to any direct action of the PPI's on the bacterium.

It seems to be well accepted that patients with duodenal or gastric ulcer will benefit from eradication of *H. pylori*. While there is no approved protocol in the USA as yet for *H. pylori* eradication, a combination of omeprazole and amoxicillin has been approved for eradication in the United Kingdom and Sweden. It seems logical that as optimal formulation is achieved for full inhibition of acid secretion by omeprazole or other PPI's, eradication regimens will become shorter and more effective in ulcer patients and that a combination of antibiotic with a PPI will become the treatment of choice.

(iii) Triple/quadruple therapy

Another therapeutic approach to *H. pylori* eradication is triple therapy, often in combination with an anti-secretory drug (i.e., quadruple therapy). Triple therapy is a combination of amoxicillin or tetracycline (qid), metronidazole (tid) and bismuth (qid), requiring the taking of at least 11 or more tablets per day (25). The organism develops resistance to metronidazole and the therapeutic regimen is complicated, suggesting that compliance and tolerability may be a problem in practice. Side effects of sore mouth, nausea and diarrhea have been reported in about 30% of patients. Studies are also under way adding the H_2 receptor antagonist ranitidine to the above regimen, making this quadruple therapy. Given the considerations regarding the bacterial environment as determining its response to antibiotics, and the relative inefficacy of H_2 receptor antagonists, it seems likely that this addition does not contribute to eradication, but contributes only to healing (25,26). Although cumbersome, it is generally agreed that triple therapy is effective in *H. pylori* eradication.

FIG. 40. *A model illustrating the concept that* H. pylori *resides on the surface of the gastric epithelium, but the pH is too low for growth. With the administration of omeprazole, the surface pH elevates to allow multiplication of the organism with, now, effectiveness of amoxicillin (a growth-dependent antibiotic) in killing the bacterium.*

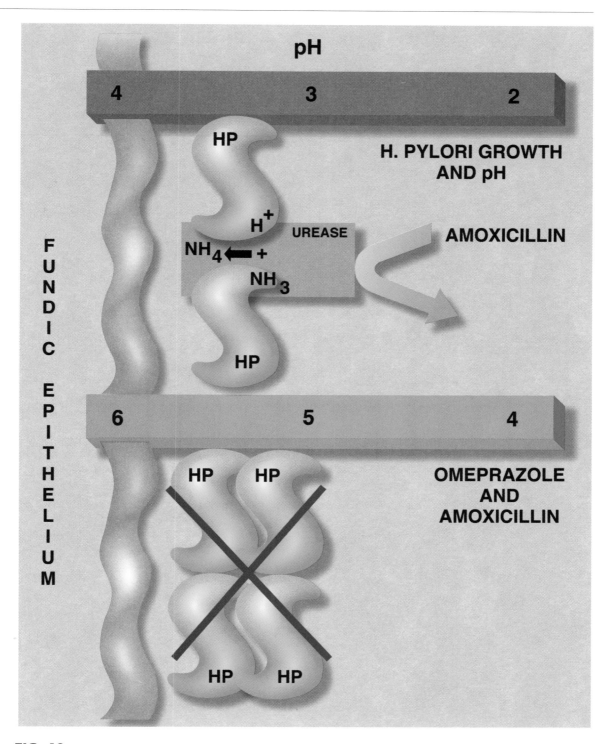

FIG. 40

(iv) Current recommendations

It would seem that therapeutic regimens designed to simultaneously heal the ulcer and eradicate *H. pylori* will become the recommended treatment for either gastric (non-NSAID) or duodenal ulcer patients in the future. These dual, triple or quadruple combinations will provide both therapeutic and economic benefit, since with eradication, maintenance therapy with drugs for duodenal and gastric ulcer appears to be no longer required. This is the conclusion reached by a recent consensus meeting at the National Institutes of Health (27).

The recommendation of the working party discussed in reference 23 or the consensus statement from the NIH panel is that there is no rationale as yet for *H. pylori* eradication in non-ulcer patients except under controlled clinical trial conditions (23).

However, it may become desirable to treat patients prospectively and eradicate *H. pylori* in the absence of symptomatic peptic ulcer disease. This approach will depend on proof of an association between gastritis and infection, as well as proof of the association between atrophic gastritis and neoplasia (12). In the absence of peptic ulcer disease, monotherapy would be desirable, but no drug has as yet demonstrated monotherapeutic efficacy. It remains a future discovery.

REFERENCES

1. Sanders M.J., Ayalon A., Roll M., and Soll A.H.: The apical surface of canine chief cell monolayers resists H+ back-diffusion. Nature 313, 52, 1985.

2. Silen W.: Gastric mucosal defense and repair. In, Johnson LR, ed. Physiology of the gastrointestinal tract. 2nd. edition, Vol 2, p 1055. Raven Press, New York, 1987.

3. Quigley E.M., and Turnberg L.A.: pH of the microclimate lining human gastric duodenal mucosa in vivo. Studies in control subjects and in duodenal ulcer patients. Gastroenterology 92, 1876, 1987.

4. Carson D.Y., Strom B.L., Morse M.L., et al.: The relative gastrointestinal toxicity of the nonsteroidal anti-inflammatory drugs. Arch. Int. Med. 147, 1054, 1987.

5. Marshall B.: Unidentified curved bacilli on gastric epithelium in active chronic gastritis. Lancet i,1273, 1983.

6. Peterson W.L.: Helicobacter pylori and peptic ulcer disease. N. Eng. J. Med. 324, 1043, 1990.

7. Bell N.J.V., Burget D., Howden C.W., Wilkinson J., and R.H. Hunt.: Appropriate acid suppression for the management of gastroesophageal reflux disease. Digestion 51, 59, 1992.

8. McCarthy D.M.: Sucralfate. N. Eng. J. Med. 325, 1017, 1991.

9. Burget D.W., Chiverton S.G., and R.H. Hunt.: Is there an optimal degree of acid suppression for healing of duodenal ulcers? Gastroenterology 99, 349, 1990.

10. Walt R.P.: Misoprostol for the treatment of peptic ulcer and anti-inflammatory drug induced gastroduodenal ulceration. NEJM 327. 1575, 1991.

11. Blaser M.J.: Hypothesis on the pathogenesis and natural history of Helicobacter pylori induced inflammation. Gastroenterology 102, 720, 1992.

12. Parsonnet J., Friedman G.D., Vandersteed D.P., et al.: H. pylori infection and the risk of gastric cancer. N. Eng. J. Med. 325, 1131, 1991.

13. Malfertheimer P., et al. Helicobacter pylori, gastritis, and peptic ulcer. Springer Verlag, Berlin, Germany 1990.

14. Schade C., Flemstrom G., and Holm L. Hydrogen ion concentration in the mucus layer on top of acid-stimulated and -inhibited rat gastric mucosa. Gastroenterology 107, 180, 1994

15. Tsuda M., Karita M., Morshed M.G., Okita K., and Nakazawa T. A.: Urease-negative mutant of Helicobacter pylori constructed by allelic exchange mutagenesis lacks the ability to colonize the nude mouse stomach. Infect. Immun. 62 3586, 1994

16. Matin A.: Bioenergetic parameters and transport in obligate acidophiles. Biochim. Biophys. Acta 1018, 267, 1990

17. Chiba N., Rao B.V., Rademaker J.W., and Hunt R.H.: Meta-analysis of the efficacy of antibiotic therapy in eradicating H. Pylori. Am. J. Gastroenterol. 87, 1716, 1992.

18. Blaser M.J.: Gastric Campylobacter-like organisms, gastritis, and peptic ulcer disease. Gastroenterology 93, 371, 1987.

19. Graham D.Y.: Helicobacter, its epidemiology and its role in duodenal ulcer disease. J. Gastroenterol. Hepatol. 6, 105, 1991.

20. Marshall B.J. Goodwin C.S. Warren J.R. et al.: Prospective double blind trial of duodenal ulcer relapse after eradication of Campylobacter pylori. Lancet 2,1437–1482,1990.

21. Bayerdoerffer E., Mannes G.A., Sommer A., Hoechter W., Weingart J., Hatz R., Lehn N., Ruckdeschel G., Dirschedl P., and Stolte M.: High dose omeprazole treatment combined with amoxicillin eradicates Helicobacter pylori. Eur. J. Gastroenterol. Hepatol. 4, 697, 1992.

22. Labenz J., Gyenes E., Ruehl G.H., and Boersch G.: Omeprazole plus amoxicillin. Efficacy of various treatments regimens to eradicate Helicobacter pylori. Am. J. Gastroenterol. 88, 491, 1992.

23. Unge P., Gad A., Erkisson K., Bergman,B., Carling L., Ekstrom P., Glise H., Gnarpe H., Junghard O., Lindhomer, C., Sandzen B., Strandberg L., Stuberrod A. and Wewadt L.: Eur. J. Gastroenterol Hepatol. 5,325, 1993.

24. Tytgat GNJ, Lee A, Graham DY, Dixon MF, and Rokkas T.: The role of infectious agents in peptic ulcer disease. Gastroenterol. Int. 6,76,1993.

25. Mohamed H, Chiba N, Wilkinson J, and Hunt R.: Eradication of helicobacter pylori, a metaanalysis. Gastroenterology 107, 1994

26. Hentschel, E, Brandstatter, G, Dragosics, B., Hirschl A.M., Nemec, H., Schutze, K., Taufer, M. and Wurzer, H.: Effect of ranitidine and amoxicillin plus metronidazole on the eradication of helicobacter pylori and the recurrence of duodenal ulcer. N. Eng. J. Med. 328, 308 1993.

27. NIH Consensus Development Panel on Helicobacter pylori in Peptic Ulcer Disease NIH Consensus Conference.: Helicobacter pylori in peptic ulcer disease. JAMA 272, 65, 1994.

Our thanks are due especially to Dr Herbert Helander and to Dr Juan Lechago for supplying the electron micrographs that we colorized, ars gratia artis, for this book.

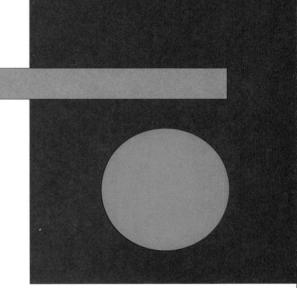

Index